How to Manage
Day and Night Wetting in Children

Dr. Wm. Lane M. Robson

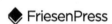 FriesenPress

One Printers Way
Altona, MB R0G 0B0
Canada

www.friesenpress.com

ISBN
978-1-03-913615-1 (Hardcover)
978-1-03-913614-4(Paperback)
978-1-03-913616-8 (eBook)

1. HEALTH & FITNESS, CHILDREN'S HEALTH

Distributed to the trade by The Ingram Book Company

Table of Contents

Author's Note

For the last fifteen years, I devoted my clinical work exclusively to voiding problems in children. When you work all day, every day in one narrow field, you learn things.

The basic non-invasive tools necessary to understand voiding problems in children include a meticulous history to identify and clarify symptoms, focused physical examination, pre- and post-void ultrasound of the bladder and rectum, uroflow study, and urinalysis.

Three decisions made a big difference in my learning journey. First, I decided to let the history from the mother and the child guide my learning. I spent two hours with the initial consultation to hear the story and to ask and answer questions. I spent an hour with each follow-up session. Based on these discussions, I built a database of more than three thousand children. Second, I decided not to use conventional diagnosis definitions of voiding problems. I did not "label" a child with a diagnosis such as "overactive bladder." Rather, I decided to think and talk about problems based on the presenting symptoms (frequency, urgency, daytime wetting, nighttime wetting). Third, I purchased an ultrasound and used this to assess the bladder and rectum in every child with every visit. I taught myself how to use the ultrasound. There was minimal data in the medical literature on even the basic measurements available to understand bladder and rectal health and function in children. I established my own normal ranges for bladder wall thickness in the anterior and posterior views, transverse rectal diameter under a full and empty bladder, and post-void residual volume. I learned how the uroflow curve changes as bladder pressure increases in children who hold the urine past full. This was a grand adventure. I spent over a decade going where no pediatric nephrologist had gone before.

With experience, I learned the rhythm of basic voiding symptoms. Common patterns emerged. My explanations started to resonate more and more with the parents. This happens when the explanations for the patterns make sense.

The explanations help parents understand complex neurobehaviour processes. Perhaps my explanations will stand the test of time. In due course, other clinicians will likely provide better clarity.

Acknowledgement

Bill Warzak, Ph.D. Professor of Psychology at the University of Wisconsin is a long-time friend and professional colleague. Bill and I served on the National Kidney Foundation Committee on Bedwetting. Bill is a first-class researcher, clinician, and teacher. His advice improved this book. Thank you, Bill.

Daytime Voiding Problems

Occam's Razor – The simplest explanation is usually the best. In the majority of children, there are only two factors to consider in voiding problems.

1. The Poop Wall – The role of bowel health.

2. Neurobiology – The role of the frontal lobes and the limbic system.

Of these, the Poop Wall comes first. Poop pressing into the bladder at the bottom of a small pelvis reduces the size of the bladder. The neurobiology is the response to a small bladder.

Voiding problems are rarely due to a physical problem. A careful history, focused physical examination, ultrasound of the bladder and rectum, uroflow study, and urinalysis are sufficient to confirm that a physical problem is not present.

Bladder infection is another cause of a small bladder that is especially common in girls. The urine should be checked several times in girls.

The Poop Wall – The Role of Bowel Health

Why doesn't every doctor who treats voiding problems in children talk about bowel health?

The relationship of bowel health to bladder function is a recent discovery. The relationship came to my attention in the eighties. I read an article that linked constipation with bladder problems. My personal clinical research, published in 1999 in Pediatrics, the official journal of the American Pediatric Association, supported the association. Since then, I've focused on the role of bowel health in voiding problems.

Another reason for the relative neglect of this association is the training and experience of the specialists who care for children with voiding problems. Paediatric Urology and Paediatric Nephrology doctors are experts in the urinary tract but not in the gastrointestinal tract. This changes how they think about a problem.

A third reason is most doctors don't usually spend enough time with families or ask the right questions.

Before a family arrives at my clinic, the mother is requested to fill out a voiding and poop questionnaire. This provides a data base. The questionnaire introduces the topics to be discussed and gets the mother thinking. One poop question is how many days in a week does your child poop? The mother is asked to circle a number from 1 to 7. The majority of mothers of school-aged children think their child poops every day. I've learned not to rely on this information. The mothers likely presume they know and don't ask their child. After their child is about six years of age, many mothers lose touch with the bowel health. The child is independent and no longer needs help to wipe. If the child does not complain about a poop problem, most mothers presume their child is a daily pooper. Rather than rely on the mother, I routinely ask the child about bowel health. By grade one a child can answer questions about how often they poop. This is my typical dialogue with a six-year-old boy. *Bobby, I'd like to ask you a question about your poop.* I let Bobby think for a moment. *Bobby, do you poop every day or are there some days you don't poop?* Bobby thinks and the most common answer is "I don't poop every day." *Bobby, that's the most common answer a boy gives me. Bobby, some boys who don't poop every day only miss one day. But some boys can go two days in a row without a poop. Do you ever go two days in a row?* If Bobby advises he can miss two days in a row I ask about three days and so on until I clarify the pattern.

What I've learned is that only about ten percent of children who come to my clinic are daily poopers. About sixty percent miss days every week but are not complaining of poop problems. The remaining thirty percent miss days and have poop symptoms (abdominal pain, difficult or painful to pass poops, poop in the pants, plugging the toilet).

There is not much room at the bottom of a pelvis. The pelvis of a newborn infant is small. Perhaps you might fit a golf ball in this tiny space. There is rapid growth in the first two years, by which time the volume might accommodate a baseball. By early elementary age the pelvis might accommodate a softball. The growth speeds up in adolescence with the pubertal growth spurt.

The funnel-shaped pelvic bones make the space narrow at the bottom. The bladder and the rectum are literally side-by-side, crammed cheek-to-jowl into the narrowest portion.

The bones of the pelvis don't move. The bladder is a muscular organ designed to squirt a liquid out a hole. The bladder is not designed to push solid poop out of the way. I call the interface between the bladder and bowel the **Poop Wall**. The Poop Wall is most prominent on the left side where the descending colon comes down beside the bladder and below where the rectum goes under the bladder.

The Poop Wall limits the size of the bladder. I use pregnancy and the effects of the growing baby on the size and control of the bladder of the mother as an analogy. Most mothers recollect the need to pee more often during pregnancy (smaller bladder volume) and urgency and dampness (less bladder control) if bathroom access is not immediately available.

Most people think of the bladder as a spherical container with curved sides. The Poop Wall is evident when you look at an ultrasound. When the child has daily poops and the stool is soft, the bladder does have a roughly spherical shape with curves. However, when the child does not poop every day and when the poop is solid, the bladder looks more like a square or rectangle. You can see solid poop pressing into the bladder, especially on the left side and below the bladder.

When the bladder has a curve the lowest part of the bladder looks like a smile-emoticon. Conversely when there is no curve and the rectal poop presses into the bladder, the appearance looks like a frown-emoticon.

I talk about bowel health in every child with every visit. I also do an ultrasound of the pelvis with every visit. This allows me to see the correlation between the symptoms and the bowel-bladder interface. Seeing is believing. Every day I see how the Poop Wall correlates with the symptoms in a child. Most of my peers, the paediatric urology and nephrology doctors who manage voiding problems, don't do their own ultrasounds. They send a child to the diagnostic imaging department. A technician does the ultrasound. Then, a diagnostic imaging doctor interprets the images and sends a report to the paediatric urologist or nephrologist. The report arrives days or weeks later. By eliminating the technician and ultrasound doctor, I gain an immediate and intimate understanding of the relationship between symptoms and the ultrasound images.

Bowel health has a major impact on bladder function. This doesn't mean all children with bladder problems have constipation. I don't prefer to use the word constipation. There are various definitions of constipation, too much misinformation, and the word comes with emotional baggage for some parents. Rather I prefer to think of bowel health as either **Bladder-Friendly** ☺ or **Not-Bladder-Friendly** ☹. Only about a third of the children in my clinic qualify for a diagnosis of constipation.

When the bowel health is not-bladder-friendly during early infancy before toilet training, the rectum takes up the space at the bottom of the pelvis and the bladder is obliged to expand up and out of the pelvis. In some children with poor bowel health from early infancy there is so much poop at the bottom of the pelvis the bladder takes on a tubular shape. On the ultrasound the tube-shaped bladder courses from the bottom of the pelvis just under the abdominal wall to the brim of the pelvis. Once free of the bony constraints the bladder expands to a spherical shape. On the ultrasound this looks like a mushroom on top of a narrow stalk. This often presents as prominence in the lower abdomen, much like a "baby bump."

When bowel health that is not-bladder-friendly develops after toilet training, the relatively larger size of the pelvis is such that the bladder is less often pushed up and out of the pelvis by hard stool. More often the bladder is "trapped" at the bottom.

Before a child starts to walk, infants are usually lying down and this posture likely favours whether the bladder can be pushed out of the pelvis. After the child starts to walk, the upright posture allows the poop to settle on the bladder and this likely favours "trapping" the bladder at the bottom.

Bladder size differs in children depending on the age when the child developed bowel health that is not-bladder-friendly. Bladder size is always compromised by solid stool in a small pelvis, but the bladders that are pushed up and out of the pelvis in early infancy hold more than the bladders that were trapped after toilet training. By grade one, the bladder size in children who developed not-bladder-friendly bowel health in early infancy is often about fifty to seventy-five percent of average. This is enough to allow night dryness in some children. Conversely, a child with not-bladder-friendly bowel health from toilet training might have a bladder size about twenty-five to fifty percent of average by grade one. This is not enough to allow night dryness.

The transverse rectal diameter under the full and the empty bladder is an index of bowel health. Under the full bladder in a child with optimal bowel health the transverse rectal diameter should be less than twenty-five millimeters. The diameter just above the rectum under the empty bladder should be less than fifteen millimeters. Diameters wider than these measurements imply the child does not poop ever day or that the child does not empty when they poop, or both. The most common measurements in children who attend my clinic are in the thirty- to forty-millimeter range in a child with a full bladder, but I also see children with measurements in the fifty-millimeter range. The widest transverse rectal diameter I ever measured is ninety millimeters! Mothers of children with bowel health symptoms often remark about how wide the poop looks. A common comment is, "I don't know how that came out," or "The poop is adult size." The mothers commonly talk about two-inch poops (size of a baseball) and sometimes three-inch poops (softball). These descriptions correlate with the transverse rectal diameter. The rectum should be a triangle at the bottom (conforms to the shape of pelvis) and a circle or oval under the full bladder. A "floppy" rectum that does not conform to a tight circle or oval implies the pressure in the rectum has been chronically elevated and for sufficient time for the muscle tone in the rectum to be compromised. Once rectal tone is compromised, this increases the challenge to achieve and sustain bladder-friendly bowel health.

Once I understood the important role of Poop Wall I needed to learn how to manage bowel health. Initially I sent children to a Paediatric Gastroenterologist. This didn't work. The clinical goals of a Paediatric Gastroenterologist are different than mine. I want to make the bladder happy. Paediatric Gastroenterology doctors want to make constipation symptoms go away. As well, the waiting times to see these doctors was often months. I needed to manage the bowel health on my own and in a timely manner. I developed a management philosophy to achieve **Bladder-Friendly Bowel Health**.

How Does Not-Bladder-Friendly Bowel Health Develop?

Children learn to hold their poop in and postpone the need to poop. Every not-bladder-friendly bowel health situation starts with holding the poop in. A child can learn to hold in the poop from the first week of life. Holding the poop in is not a "conscious" process for infants and toddlers. Likely what happens is the poop firms up and is uncomfortable to pass. The infant doesn't like the discomfort. Next time the poop arrives in the rectum, rather than relaxing and letting the poop out, the infant tenses the pelvic floor muscles to slow down or stop the poop to avoid the discomfort. If the poop is regularly uncomfortable to pass, the default state for the child is to routinely hold in the poop. This happens automatically without "conscious" thought. I point this out to parents because some believe the child holds in the poop purposefully. If a parent believes this, the parent might judge the child, and the parent might discipline the child. The child does not hold the poop in in a "conscious" purposeful fashion. The child learns to hold the poop in to avoid discomfort. Eventually this becomes automatic, like breathing. The child should not be judged or disciplined for something they don't realize they are doing.

Most breastfed infants poop multiple times a day, usually after a feeding. The typical pattern is feed then poop, feed then poop, and so on. This normal pattern is how poop is meant to come out. The food lands in the stomach and this initiates the gastro-colic (stomach-colon) reflex. The muscles in the bowel wall automatic contract to push poop in the intestine along. This makes perfect sense. When we eat, the intestines need to push the poop along to make room for the ingested food in the stomach that will soon arrive in the intestine. There is no reason why an older child or adult should not have a poop after each meal and some do. This isn't common but happens.

Poop inevitably firms up from the loose breast milk poops. The common times for this to happen are when solids are added or when the child is weaned to cow's milk. Poop firms up with any situation that causes dehydration. Poor feeding due to a respiratory illness is a common cause of dehydration. Dehydration due to stomach flu with diarrhea often results in paradoxical constipation after the diarrhea settles. Dehydration due to too much sun on a winter vacation is another common scenario. Poops usually firm up after routine childhood operations due to either dehydration or the effect of pain medication on bowel motility. Regardless of what causes the firm poop, the pattern changes. The number of poops each day decrease and the pattern gets random. Problems start when the poop gets firm enough to be uncomfortable and the child learns to hold the poop in. The pattern changes to a random later-in-the-day pattern and then to missed days.

I ask parents how they know that their child pooped as an infant. Some say smell. Others report they routinely check at expected times after feeding. Others report a red face, grunting, pushing, or other body language clues that imply the poop is uncomfortable to pass. This is the start of the not-bladder-friendly bowel health problem.

Tip-toe walking is a hold-the-poop-in behaviour. The pelvic floor muscles are tense when a child walks on their tip-toes. Some parents report their child braces against a chair or a table when they poop. Most parents presume the child does this to help the poop come out. Most of the bracing postures are actually learned responses to hold the poop in! The child is conflicted. The body knows the poop needs to come out but the memory of the discomfort is enough for the child to try to stop or at least slow down the poop.

Some parents report their infant went multiple days or a week without a poop. Most parents get worried in this situation and consult their doctor or a public health nurse. There is a myth that it is "normal" for a breast fed baby to miss a week of poops. The word "common" is a much better way to describe this. Missing multiple days or a week is not normal. Missing days is common but never normal.

When the pressure of stool in the rectum is high and when a child loses touch with the signals of the need to poop, the stool sneaks out into the clothes. Soiling is the word I use for poop accidents. Another word is encopresis.

Bowel health changes day by day and week by week in children. Children poop on some days but not on other days. Some mothers report that pee and poop accidents come together in waves or spurts. These words are great metaphors for the problems. Most parents use these words without realizing the significance. Waves are wetting episodes. Spurts are soiling episodes. When the child is in a wave or a spurt the bowel health is worse. When the bowel health is worse there is a higher pressure in the rectum and the poop sneaks out. When the bowel health is worse there is a higher pressure on the bladder and the pee sneaks out. Pee and poop accidents coming together in waves or spurts is a great illustration of the intimate relationship between the bladder and the bowel. Most parents don't recognize the relationship until I point this out. Learning this is important. Once they can appreciate the relationship between poop and pee, they understand what needs to be done to solve the problem.

Children with autism are especially prone to hold in their poop. The poop gets harder and wider and more difficult to pass. When the poop gets "stuck" some children with autism use their finger to help remove the piece of poop that is blocking the exit. Once they have poop on their fingers, they usually wipe the poop on the nearest available surface which is a wall or toilet seat. This makes a real mess and is often misinterpreted by the parents and physicians. This is not a "behavioural" problem. This is the way a child with autism solves the "stuck-poop" problem. This is a practical solution. I've helped a lot of mothers of children with autism get past the poop-on-the-wall-symptom with this explanation.

The Three Goals of Bladder-Friendly Bowel Health

1. Poop every morning after breakfast before the child leaves home for daycare or for school.

2. Empty well with every poop.

3. Poop that is soft enough for the bladder to push out of the way.

Poop every morning after breakfast before the child leaves home for daycare or for school

Achieving this goal insures the child will attend school with more space for the bladder at the bottom of the pelvis and a rectum that is not loaded under pressure.

A bladder that will hold more while the child is at school has many practical advantages. The child will need to pee less often. The child will not need to ask the teacher for permission to leave class as often. The child will not need to interrupt class work or play activities as often. The child will be more inclined to drink more because they don't need to pee as often. The child with daytime wetting will have less risk of wetting. In a more complicated sense, and not something proven, but something I believe likely, the volume a child practices peeing during the day sets the volume the bladder empties at night. This is important in children who either wake up to pee (nocturia) or wet the bed.

The first morning poop is even more essential when poop accidents are part of the problem. **The solution to soiling is a morning poop.** If the child poops in the morning, the pressure in the rectum is reduced, and the risk of poop accident later in the day is low.

Five things are necessary to achieve a morning poop

1. Both the child and mother need to have enough time to work on the morning routine. A minimum of one hour is necessary from the time the child wakes up until they leave the house for daycare or for school. Mornings are rushed in many families. I did a survey and found that most children have only 45 minutes from wake up to leave

for school. Amazingly I learned of families who only had twenty minutes from waking to leaving! These children often eat their breakfast in the car or on the bus. Homes are rushed when there are lots of children in the home, especially pre-school children. Most families will need to get their child up at least fifteen minutes earlier to have enough time. This means getting the child to bed fifteen minutes earlier. The mother needs to plan her personal bedtime to insure she is rested and up early enough to accomplish the myriad of important tasks necessary for a mother to get the family up and on their way for the day.

2. The child needs to routinely sit on the toilet after breakfast. Breakfast should be planned earlier after waking rather than closer to departure time. The child needs to sit for ten minutes, by the clock, **whether they feel like they need to poop or not**. The child will not feel like they need to poop at the start and this might confuse the child. From the perspective of a young child, if they don't feel like they need to poop, there is no poop there, so why sit? The mother needs to finesse the cooperation of the child.

3. The mother needs to personally supervise the child while sitting in the bathroom. I designate the mother as the **Personal Poop Trainer Mom.** She should be in the room with the child. This is very important at the front end of the project. This is especially important for pre-school and early elementary-aged children. Once the skill set is achieved, this is less important. One-to-one supervision is important for several reasons. This is a solidarity principle. The presence of the mother is a strong statement that the child is not alone, that the mother is there to help and support, that they are a team. Most younger children view the presence of the mother as a reward and this is a good way to finesse compliance. One-on-one time with a mother is a special time when the mother does not divide her attention between the siblings. Supervision is necessary to insure the child does sit and ensures the mother will see the poop.

4. Make the ten minutes enjoyable. The mother and child can talk, read, or watch a video together.

5. Be patient. Morning poops might take a few months to settle in. This much time is necessary because achieving the poop softness necessary for a morning poop takes time and should not be rushed.

If the child does not poop after sitting for ten minutes, the parent should thank the child for sitting. Until the child is at least a daily pooper, the parent should structure sitting on the toilet after lunch on days the child is home, after the snack when the child arrives home after school, and after supper. Until the child is a daily pooper, the parent should structure sitting after as many meals and snacks as possible during the day.

Changing any behaviour takes time and consistency. Asking a child to sit to poop when they don't feel like they need to poop is a challenge for some parents. Parents need to offer the necessary time and consistency for the project and they need to finesse the cooperation of the child. Some parents have the time and skill set to accomplish this. Others don't. Some children are more cooperative than others. At one end of the cooperative spectrum are children who are "rule followers." At the other end of the cooperate spectrum are children who are oppositional. Progress is straightforward when the parent has the necessary time and skill set and the child cooperates. In some families the child is in cooperative mode but the parent is not able to provide the necessary structure and supervision for success. Until the child is old enough to accept responsibility on their own (usually in the last few years of elementary school), there will be slow or no progress. In other families the parent has the time and skill set but the child will not cooperate. Without cooperation by the child, there will be slow or no progress. The worst scenario is a parent who is impatient, rushed, and does not have the skill set to finesse cooperation, and an uncooperative child. This usually ends up with confrontations every morning. Confrontations are never helpful. When confrontations develop the parent should back off and let time pass. The parent should wait until the child is older, more mature, and demonstrates personal motivation for dryness. Lots of families visit my clinic, work on the recommendations, realize the challenges, back off, and return a year or two later, when circumstances are improved.

Empty well with every poop

Don't take emptying for granted. The Poop Wall persists if the rectum doesn't empty.

There are four basic principles to achieve good emptying.

1. Sit with a posture that relaxes the pelvic floor muscles.

2. Consciously relax while sitting with the correct posture.

3. Don't rush. Take your time.

4. Don't push.

Sit with a posture that relaxes the pelvic floor muscles

The pelvic floor muscles are the muscles around the bum hole. The majority of the children in my clinic regularly hold their pee and their poop past full. This means they regularly "exercise" their pelvic floor muscles. This makes the pelvic floor muscles chronically tense. Unless these muscles relax, the poop will not come out or will be slow to empty. Unless these muscles relax the emptying will be compromised. In children who chronically keep their pelvic floor muscles tense to hold in pee and poop, I often see spontaneous contractions of the pelvic floor muscles when I perform a pelvic ultrasound.

Some of the children in my clinic have memories of painful bowel movements. These children usually keep the pelvic floor muscles tense during a poop to minimize the risk of remembered pain. This is counter-productive but the child does not realize they are doing this. The child is in automatic hold-the-poop-in mode.

The correct posture to relax the pelvic floor muscles is to emulate the squat. Before modern bathrooms, people squatted in designated poop places. This still happens in communities without modern plumbing. A squat naturally relaxes the pelvic floor muscles. The squat is the natural posture to poop, to pee, and for a woman to deliver a baby.

To emulate a squat there are three principles.

1. Sit in the middle of the toilet. Until the age of about 6 years most children need an over the toilet seat to achieve this. The child should not need to perch forward or hold themselves up with their hands on the toilet seat to avoid falling in. The child should not sink into the toilet.

2. The pants and the underwear should be off so the knees relax shoulder-width apart.

3. **The feet including the heels MUST be flat** on either the ground or a footstool. Until the age of about 6 years, most children need a footstool.

The Personal Poop Trainer Mom needs to supervise these principles and ensure the child practices the principles.

Periodically a mother tells me their pre-school child squats standing on the toilet seat to poop. These children impress me. They have a history of difficulties pooping and they independently learn that if they squat standing on the toilet seat, the poop comes out easier. How did they learn this? My guess is that while struggling to poop they experimented with a variety of maneuvers to help the poop come out. First, they learned that if they bring their thighs up this helps. Then they learned that if they flatten their feet this helps. Finally, they put the behaviours together and learn to squat standing on the toilet seat. Amazing! These children have precocious problem-solving abilities.

Tip-toe walking in a toddler is a hold-the-poop-in posture. Walking on tip-toes is the opposite of a squat. Tip-toe walking ensures tense pelvic floor muscles. Flat heels are essential to relax the pelvic floor muscles. If you want to understand this personally, the next time you pass a pasty log, suddenly lift your heels off the floor and go up on your tip-toes. You will feel the poop slow down. Same thing if you suddenly put your knees together. Posture is very important.

Consciously relax while sitting with the correct posture

Just because you sit with the optimal posture does not guarantee that the pelvic floor muscles will relax. The child must consciously relax while in the optimal posture. Many children have memories of painful, difficult to pass poops and they do not relax while sitting on the toilet. They need to learn to relax.

I ask the Personal Poop Trainer Mom to coach their child in some deep breathing exercises while sitting on the toilet. My teaching dialogue goes something like this. "Breathe in. Breathe out. Big breath in. Big breath out. Bigger breath in. Bigger breath out. Feel your body relax as you breath out."

Some children are busy. They don't sit still. The Personal Poop Trainer Mom needs to find ways to finesse relaxation in a busy child. Most will settle if you offer them electronics. This is a good time for electronics. Use electronics as a reward for compliance with the principles. Some are so pre-occupied with the electronics the poop comes out and the child does not realize they pooped!

Don't rush. Take your time

I recommend ten minutes sitting on the toilet even if you don't feel the need to poop. If the child doesn't poop, thank the child for cooperating. Then try again after lunch if the child is home for the day, or after school or supper. If the child does poop, always wait a minute or two after the poop stops coming out in case there is a following poop to come.

Don't push

Pushing compromises emptying. When you push, both the abdominal and pelvic floor muscles get tense. When the pelvic floor muscles get tense the poop slows down. When you push, the tense pelvic floor muscles can pinch off the poop. One piece falls in the toilet. The higher-up piece is still in the rectum. If the child does not relax, the following piece might not come out. The Personal Poop Trainer Mom needs to supervise this principle. The poop should come out naturally. Only the muscles in the bowel wall should do the pushing. Pushing is common at the start because the poop is not soft. As the poop slowly softens, pushing should be discouraged.

Poop soft enough for the bladder to push out of the way

Success with bladder-friendly bowel health is all about soft poop. My definition of soft poop is different than the Pediatric

Gastroenterology specialists. They use the Bristol Stool Scale. I don't. My definition of soft poop is about process and outcome, not about shape and consistency.

If the poop is soft enough,

1. The poop comes out without pushing when the child sits after breakfast.

2. The child starts to have a second poop each day, usually after lunch on a weekend, or after school or supper on a school day.

3. The child no longer has voiding urgency. There is no rush to get to the bathroom. The poop wall is gone. The bladder pushes through the poop. The child has more time to get to the bathroom.

4. The child can appreciate the bladder is getting bigger. They are drinking more but go longer between voids. The pee takes longer to come out (more noticeable with the first morning void). The parents need to stop less often on road trips.

Conversely, if the poop is not soft enough,

1. The child does not poop every day

2. The child is not pooping routinely in the morning after breakfast.

3. The child still has urgency when they go to the bathroom.

4. The child is still peeing frequently or wetting by day.

When an elementary-aged child returns for follow up after working for several months on bladder-friendly bowel health I ask the child some specific questions. *Bobby, does your bladder feel different now compared to before?* Some reply, "Yes," and I respond, *How does your bladder feel different?* The various answers I hope to hear include "better" and "bigger." Most answer "I don't know," to which I respond, *Bobby, when you go pee now do you have more time to get to the bathroom or less time?* The answer I hope to hear is "more time." A "better" "bigger" or "more time" answer confirms the bowel health has improved and is now more bladder friendly and the Poop Wall has started to resolve.

At the follow up visit I ask the parents if they think the bladder is bigger. When a parent answers "Yes" I ask them to give me an example that proves the bladder is bigger. The answers I hope to hear include, "His pee volumes are bigger," "He goes longer between voids but is drinking more," and "We don't need to stop as often on road trips."

Soft poop is softer than paste, breaks apart, but is not liquid. You can control soft poop. To achieve soft poop there are three ingredients.

1. Water

2. Natural fibre in the diet

3. Poop Softener

All three are necessary. **Water is the most important** because natural fibre and the stool softener I recommend is not effective if there is not enough water in the body.

Less than optimal hydration is always part of the problem. The most common drinking pattern in a school age child with day or night wetting is a variation of the following. The child does not drink much at breakfast, perhaps just milk on cereal. The child does not drink much at school, perhaps a juice box at lunch, but often only a few trips to the water fountain. If they take a water bottle, the bottle comes home close to full. Children don't drink because a small bladder means they need to leave class to pee or might suffer daytime wetting if this is part of the problem. Less commonly, the parents, caregivers, and school teachers limit fluid intake during the school day as their response to voiding frequently or daytime wetting. The child finishes their school day dehydrated and thirsty and the biggest drink of the day is when they arrive home. Parents who pick up their child often remark the child starts to guzzle from their water bottle as soon as they get in the car. The child might drink again before supper and then has another big drink at supper because they are still behind on their hydration. After supper, parents of a child with bedwetting commonly limit fluids (wrong but common). The child doesn't drink while asleep. This drinking pattern results in satisfactory hydration for only about four hours in the entire day from home time to supper time! This hydration pattern guarantees a dehydrated child and solid, hard or pasty poop in a random later-in-the-day pattern, and missed days. This pattern also guarantees the kidneys will make the majority of the pee overnight.

Most parents believe their child is drinking lots but they aren't. I think the parent believes the child is drinking lots because of the substantial thirst-generated drinking from after school to supper time. It is important for parents to realize that a thirsty child is dehydrated.

I recommend that a child wake up and immediately start to hydrate. Everyone wakes up dehydrated because we don't drink while we sleep. The child needs to **wake up and get caught up** with their hydration before lunch. The child should literally take a drink as soon as they wake up. The mother should place a glass of fresh water by the bedside before the child wakes up.

A child can usually drink about 30 ml of water per year of age before they start to make much pee. Getting caught up doesn't result in pee frequency or daytime wetting. The body doesn't use the catch-up hydration to make pee but rather uses the water to replenish hydration in various parts of the body. After the hydration in the child is caught up, the kidneys will start to make pee, the bladder will fill up, and the child will need to pee as often as the bladder fills up.

Children who take a long bus ride to school need to have their hydration managed to avoid pee frequency or daytime wetting during the time when no bathroom is available on the bus. The mother should only allow these children to drink the catch-up hydration before they leave for the bus. Families who live close to the school can work on hydration during the car ride to school and request that the child pee on arrival at school.

A child can handle peeing about four times at school. This is not too much of a bother. A child can pee this often and still learn and socialize. When a child needs to pee more often, this becomes a problem. As such, the amount of water a child needs to learn to drink in the morning at school should **start low and go up slow**. This is very important. If the child drinks too much too soon before the bladder starts to get bigger, the child will pee too often or wet at school. This erodes compliance.

I designate the mother as the **Personal Hydration Manager Mom**. I set a goal for the amount of water a child needs to drink from the time they wake up until the school lunch break. The goal is based on the weight of the child. For the average child in early elementary the amount is 750 ml. I recommend the child start with a modest amount, say 250 ml. As the child walks out the door Mom will hand her child a bottle with the desired amount of water to finish before lunch. Every week Mom will increase the water in the bottle by 25 to 50 ml, but **only if the child is coping with the amount during the prior week**. Mom needs to talk with the child. How often did they pee during the school day? Did the teacher allow easy access to the bathroom? Did the child have urgency or dampness? If everything is ok, the mother may increase the amount. If not, the mother slows down. I call this, "sneaking up on the hydration."

At lunch the child can drink whatever their preference and then the child should "coast" in the afternoon and drink only as per thirst. Most will only drink more if they have afternoon physical education class.

After school the child should drink another 30 ml per year of age when they arrive home, again at supper, and again after supper. **I purposely want the child to drink after supper, even if they wet the bed.** Drinking after supper is an important hydration concept. Pre-school and early elementary children sleep for ten to twelve hours. During this time the child does not drink. During this time the bowel is a "reservoir" of water for the body to draw upon as necessary to satisfy water needs in other organs. The body literally sucks the water out of the bowel. The rectum has special salt and water transport receptors to accomplish this. This is why the first piece of poop to come out in the morning is always more solid than the following pieces. In a dehydrated child, more water is removed. Purposefully drinking water after supper helps to minimize the water loss in the rectum overnight.

Milk, yogurt drinks, and protein shakes do not count as hydration. I consider these liquids more like solid food. Think of these liquids as more like cheese. These liquids contain a lot of fat, protein, and carbohydrate. Digestion and the metabolic process uses up the water in these beverages.

The water bottle must be on the desk or the child will not remember to drink. The child should be coached to drink slowly at school and not guzzle the water. The teacher can help by reminding the child to drink the water and by allowing easy access to the bathroom. The basic school voiding rule is the child should **always leave class to pee and never wait for the break**. If you ask a child to wait to pee they will not drink as much.

Learning to hydrate in the mornings at school, when the mother is not around to supervise, is the hardest behaviour to achieve. When you improve the hydration slowly and methodically, the child can achieve the hydration goal in about three months. Some children will not drink in the morning at school, will "remember" to drink to comply with the mother's request, and will guzzle the water at the end of the school day. This is not helpful. The child needs to learn to slowly reach the hydration goal before lunch.

The Personal Hydration Manager Mom needs to finesse cooperation. They should talk about this every day when the child arrives home from school and once a week when they make the decision whether to increase the water for the next week. They should make this a game with rewards. The parent should engage the school teacher in this project. Some teachers have the time and inclination to remind the child to drink the water before lunch.

A child needs to pee at my clinic so I can do the pre- and post-void ultrasound, the uroflow test, and check the urine under the microscope. Since most of the children are chronically dehydrated, unless they drink water at my office, they might not pee. So, I encourage children to drink water at my clinic. Most cooperate. Occasionally a child drinks enough for the urine colour to change from dark yellow (dehydrated) to clear (hydrated). Some observant children remark, "There's something wrong with my urine! It looks like water!" Children who make these comments are observant but have never been hydrated. I teach we should all drink enough in the morning for the urine to be clear sometime before lunch.

Natural Fibre in the Diet

Natural fibre in the diet is important. I ask the mother to work on fibre but rely on the stool softener. The mother needs to work on fibre because the child will eventually stop the stool softener and if the natural fibre in the diet has not improved, the bowel health will get worse.

The common sources of natural fibre are fruits and vegetables, brown grains, and beans and lentils. There is no fibre in meat, eggs, or dairy. Some children eat predominantly meat, eggs, and dairy. They need more poop softener and a longer time to change their dietary preferences. Some children naturally take more fibre and need less poop softener.

Many mothers presume the poop is soft enough because the family is vegetarian or the mother is a nutrition specialist and works at fibre. The most common reason why children in these families still have solid hard or pasty poop is the lack of good hydration.

I recommend mothers learn about the grams of fibre in the diet of their child. This requires study of the ingredient label on the package. Pre-school children need about 20 grams of fibre a day. Elementary-aged children need about 25 grams. After the age of ten years, a child needs 30 grams.

Stool Softener

I recommend a poop softener in every child with voiding problems. Early in my career I tried to achieve soft poop with only fibre and water, and this was difficult for the majority of children. I learned to accept the need for the softener and I learned how to use the softener.

The stool softener I recommend is polyethylene glycol (PEG). This is sold under a variety of trade names. Restoralax and Lax A Day in Canada. Costco has their own brand (Clearalax). Miralax in the United States. All these products contain the same chemical. PEG is sold without a prescription, which implies the regulatory agencies in Canada and the United States consider the chemical safe for over-the-counter purchase.

PEG is a white powder. This inorganic chemical has the important ability to attract and hold water around the molecule. This is how the softener makes the poop soft. It's all about the water. Natural fibre attracts and holds water in a similar fashion. I prefer PEG to other poop softeners because the chemical acts in a natural manner like fibre. The white powder is colourless and tasteless. You mix the powder in water, or whatever the child drinks.

I tell the mothers, **Do Not Follow the Package Instructions**. The package instructions are for adults and to cleanse the bowel. I am not trying to cleanse the bowel and I only see children. My goal is to slowly, methodically, improve poop softness so the bladder can learn to hold more urine and so the child has more time to get to the bathroom. I ask the mothers to **start low and go up slow**. This is the same rule as with hydration. The Personal Poop Trainer Mom is the manager. I recommend the mother give the PEG twice a day at breakfast and supper. The softener should always be given with a meal. After all, it is the food in the meal that needs to stay soft. I want the PEG to travel with the food on the journey from the stomach to the rectum.

PEG is either not absorbed into the body or minimally absorbed. This is the explanation for the modest side effect potential. The water in the intestine will change during the intestinal journey but more water will remain with the digested food if PEG is present.

I ask the mother to start with ¼ teaspoon of PEG at breakfast and another ¼ teaspoon at supper. The mother should follow the poop pattern and increase the dose by ¼ teaspoon every week or two until the child is pooping every morning and the poop comes out without the need to push. Going this slow means the poop will not get too soft too quickly. This minimizes the risk of poop accidents. Going this slow allows the child to learn how to manage softer stool. Most elementary aged children will need about one to two teaspoons of PEG both at breakfast and at supper to achieve first morning poops. Most mothers will take two or three months to determine the correct amount necessary to achieve first morning poops.

Once the child achieves the first morning poop pattern the mother should continue with the current dose of PEG until the bladder goals are reached. This usually means dry by day and dry at night. This usually requires a child to stay on the softener for at least six months and often a year.

I ask mothers to strive for consistency with administration of the PEG. They should get into a routine and give the PEG twice a day at breakfast and supper, try not to miss dosages, and methodically increase the dosage until they achieve first morning poop success. This is a challenge for many busy mothers. This is a bigger challenge when the child lives in two homes. Coordination between caregivers in the two homes is important to achieve consistency.

I ask mothers to strive for slow methodical consistency and to try not to start and stop the PEG. Starting and stopping causes a too loose or too hard, "boom or bust" pattern. The child never really gets in good touch with the poop signals because softness changes too often or too much.

Simply put, the three most important interventions to achieve a first morning poop is to supervise sitting on the toilet every morning, to learn to hydrate in the morning, and to methodically and consistently increase the PEG until the desired softness is achieved. Of these three interventions, the easiest is to take PEG.

Mothers often return to advise the child is taking the maximum dose of PEG (two teaspoons breakfast and supper) every day, but the child is still not pooping every day. The most common reason is the lack of water. The child is not drinking enough to "activate" the PEG. Giving the PEG is easy for these mothers. Getting their child to hydrate in the morning while away at school is a far greater challenge.

Some mothers are concerned about taking the PEG. They view the PEG as a medication with the potential for side effects. They have often read something that worries them about poop softeners. There is a lot of misinformation about poop softeners. The most common is that a child will become "dependent" or "addicted" to the softener. If a child has poor bowel health and requires the softener to improve the situation and to resolve the symptoms, well and good. I'm glad the softener works. If the child successfully changes their behaviour (poops each morning, improves hydration, increases fibre), these changes are usually sufficient for the child to stop the softener. This fits for the majority of children. If the child continues to need the softener to sustain the improved bowel health, this does not mean the child is dependent or addicted, this means either the bowel health is that bad or that the morning poop pattern, the hydration, and the fibre continues to need work.

There are children with bowel health problems that cannot be cured. Sometimes bowel health can only be controlled. These children need to stay on the softener to sustain control. Constipation is a lifetime problem in children with a nerve problem from the spine to the rectum (spina bifida, traumatic injury to the spine). These children require a stool softener every day for their entire lifetime. These individuals do not usually complain about being "dependent" on the softener, they are glad they can poop.

Some mothers of children with autism are especially worried about taking PEG. These mothers read and have concerns about specific misinformation about PEG in children with autism. This is similar to the misinformation about vaccines and autism. I do my best to reassure these mothers. I respect their concerns and suggest they consider other softeners or do their best with fibre and hydration.

Reward Process not Outcome

Rewards help to encourage better outcomes. When I discuss rewards with parents, I ask them to reward process not outcome. This means I do not recommend that a parent reward day or night dryness. The child has no immediate control over these outcomes. I recommend parents reward a child for cooperating with the important process behaviours that will result in the desired outcome. A parent should reward a child for cooperating to sit on the toilet for ten minutes after breakfast. A parent should reward a child for cooperating to drink the desired amount of water in the morning before lunch. A parent should reward a child for cooperating to take the stool softener twice a day. When a child cooperates to accomplish these process behaviours, the outcome will be good. Rewards should be age-appropriate, consistent and immediate, and fit with the philosophy of rewards in the family.

Neurobiology – The Basics

The basic neural pathway is from the bladder to the spinal cord to the voiding center in the brainstem and thereafter to higher centers, which importantly include the frontal lobes and limbic system. The frontal lobes are where executive decisions are made. The frontal lobes are where impulse control is mediated. The frontal lobes are where thinking (cognition) happens. The limbic system is where memory and emotion are modulated.

From birth until toilet training, while a child is still in a daytime diaper, the signal of a full bladder is sent to the voiding center and there is an automatic signal sent back down the spinal cord to the bladder to relax the external sphincter and empty the bladder. This works perfectly for a diapered child. There is no need for higher control. That is not to say that there aren't connections up to the frontal lobes or other brain areas. The connections from the voiding center to the frontal lobes are present from birth. Sleeping newborn infants open their eyes with voiding. Many mothers know when their infant is voiding. Mothers report facial expressions and other body language clues while their child voids into a diaper.

Toilet Training

Toilet training is a cognitive process whereby a child learns to hold the pee or poop until they attend in a bathroom and pee or poop into a toilet. The bladder or bowel is no longer allowed to empty in a reflex fashion into a diaper. The child is obliged to exercise higher control over this process. The child is required to make a decision to hold the pee or poop until they attend in the bathroom to use the toilet. This decision is a frontal lobe function.

Toilet training is a process where a **parent educates a child and the child learns to hold in the pee and the poop until they reach the bathroom.** It is helpful to point this out to a parent of a child who routinely holds the pee or poop past full. Many parents don't understand why their child might hold the pee or the poop past full. Once parents recognize that toilet training is the normal starting point for a child to naturally learn to hold in the pee and the poop, parents can start to appreciate the spectrum of holding behaviours that emerge.

The average age a child in North America is toilet trained is about 2.5 years. However, children are toilet trained in other cultures as early as the first year of life. In these cultures, the usual routine is for the mother to hold their infant over a potty about half an hour or so after breast or bottle feeding. The infant pees and a cuddle is offered as a reward. The child stays dry by day. Mom is happy because her child is toilet trained by day and there is no need for the expense or bother of diapers. The baby is happy because the mother is happy. Infants can also be toilet trained at night, but usually only with a mother that sleeps close enough to their infant to recognize the nocturnal body language clues that the bladder is full. When the mother notices these body language clues and wakes and takes her infant to pee, the child can learn to be dry at night. These culture-specific toilet training practices imply a child can learn to hold the pee from the first year of life. This implies the frontal lobe function is operative for these decisions.

Holding the pee past full is likely uncommon in a diapered child. One exception is a child who experiences discomfort with voiding, as might happen with bladder infection, urethral infection, or local inflammation in the external genitalia (foreskin inflammation, vulvitis, diaper rash). These children likely learn to hold their urine past full to avoid the discomfort associated with peeing in these conditions. Holding the pee past full is accomplished by increasing the tension in the pelvic floor muscles. When an infant holds the pee or poop past full because of discomfort this likely involves signals from the hippocampus (memory) and from the limbic system (emotion, pain). The signals travel to the frontal lobes with the memory of the pain and the frontal lobes make the decision to increase the tension in the pelvic floor muscles (send signals to motor cortex area that controls pelvic floor muscles).

Unless a diapered infant experiences discomfort with voiding, there is no reason a priori for the infant to hold the pee past full at the start of toilet training and most don't in the immediate days and weeks after toilet training. During toilet training when there is no past history of discomfort with voiding, it is easy to let liquid pee flow out the urethra. This is why there are accidents at the start of toilet training. The accidents continue until the child learns to hold the pee until they reach the toilet. Toilet training is usually easier for pee.

The situation for poop is different. Episodes of discomfort with pooping are common before toilet training. When I ask a mother how she knows her diapered infant has pooped they often report body language clues that indicate discomfort with pooping. The child grunts, is red in the face, or looks in pain. When I ask these mothers about prior poop behaviour they often report the child sought out a private place for the process. This might be a corner, behind a couch, or a closet.

When a mother reports that toilet training is a "challenge" or a "struggle," this invariably means the poop is the problem and that the poop problems came before the family started toilet training. In these children, the memories of uncomfortable poops are present at the start of toilet training. These children have already learned to hold in the poop. With toilet training these children continue to hold in the poop while they assess the relative merits of the potty or toilet versus the diaper. When you already have problems pooping, the potty or the toilet might look risky to a child. Most of these children would rather poop in the diaper. At least they know what to expect in the diaper. This is a common reason why children toilet train for poop slower than for pee.

Some children are more amenable to accept the change from the diaper to the toilet. This might be a personality characteristic. If a child is not keen on "change" in general, as is the case for some children, and especially for children with autism, this might make the transition from diaper to toilet problematic. A five-year-old with autism was referred to my clinic for "toilet training" problems. From the age of four years the child told her mother when she needed to pee and Mom took her into the bathroom. She refused to pee or poop on the toilet but she did pee or poop in the bathroom while wearing a diaper. The child did not wet or soil between trips to the bathroom. This child is "toilet trained." The problem is her reluctance to accept the "change" from the diaper to the toilet. The problem developed because there is a past history of difficult to pass uncomfortable poops and the child is reluctant to accept a "change."

A common story is for mothers to report the child toilet trained for pee in a few days without any problem. However, the child is reluctant to poop on the potty. The mothers report the child refuses or is frightened. In this situation, some parents try to force their child to sit on the potty or toilet. Forcing a child is never a good strategy. The emotional responses of a child who is "forced" include anger and fear. These strong emotions will not allow a child to relax and cooperate. These strong emotions build negative memories associated with the toilet training process.

Some parents understand the reluctance of their child to use the toilet and rather than allow their child to suffer holding in the poop, they give the child a diaper to poop in. Some children ask for a diaper to poop. Either way, this is a good interim strategy. Much better to let the child poop in a diaper rather than allow the child to continue to hold in the poop, which builds up in pressure in the rectum and squishes the bladder. I regularly see children who are toilet trained for pee by day but who still use a diaper to poop until kindergarten or the early elementary years. Far better to let the poop out. The child usually arrives home from school, poops in a diaper, and then carries on with their day. The bowel health in a child who still poops every day in the diaper is always better than the bowel health of a similar aged child who poops in the toilet but who misses days.

I assessed an eleven-year-old girl with significant learning problems who was treated with an enema every day of her life from the toddler years to my assessment. The girl had toilet training problems as a toddler and the advice from her doctor was to keep her in a diaper and do an enema every day. The child eventually cooperated to pee on the toilet during the day at home and at school and kept her diaper dry between trips to the bathroom. There was never any pee or poop in the diaper. The parents and the special school caregivers accepted the need for the diaper. The parents accepted the need for the daily enemas. When I did an ultrasound of the bladder and the bowel in this girl the transverse rectal diameter and the bladder wall thickness was normal and in the range of measurement you would expect in a normal toddler who never held the pee or poop. The daily enemas protected her bladder and bowel. I certainly don't recommend daily enema therapy unless this is a last resort and I definitely don't recommend enemas for years in a child with normal nerve control of the bladder, however, much like giving a child a pull up to poop in, the enemas in this child protected the bowel and the bladder. I pointed out to the parents of this girl that she had normal bladder and bowel function and that the child was toilet trained. I stopped the diaper and enemas and the child did just fine.

Some parents report their child toilet trained for pee ok but refused to poop in the potty and instead started to poop in the overnight pull up. I consider poop in the overnight pull up to be a red flag of more serious constipation. These children really know how to hold in their poop. The poop only comes out when they are asleep (unconscious) at night.

Does the age a child is toilet trained play a role in daytime voiding problems?

Is a child who is toilet trained at one year more or less likely to have daytime voiding problems than another child who is toilet trained at two years, or three years? If the bladder size is average, which implies bladder-friendly bowel health, and if frontal lobe function is mature for age, there is not likely any difference. However, if the bowel health is not-bladder-friendly or if the frontal lobe function is less mature for age, there is likely a benefit to waiting until bowel health is improved and until a child is older and frontal lobe function is more mature.

Bowel health usually gets slowly but surely worse after toilet training

It is not a question of if the bowel health gets worse, but rather how fast and whether the child will suffer symptoms due to the change in bowel health. The bowel health gets worse for three reasons.

First, while in the diaper the child can usually adopt the optimal posture to poop. An infant lying down learns to flex the thighs at the hip. A walking infant learns to squat. Once the diaper is gone, the child is obliged to learn the optimal posture sitting on a toilet. Unless the mother arranges an over-the-toilet seat and footstool, emptying is compromised. This leads to a slow methodical deterioration in bowel health.

Second, the process of toilet training is such that children are obliged to learn to hold in the poop. If they learned this during infancy, holding is enhanced when they stop the daytime diaper. Holding in the poop leads to random patterns and missed days. Children tend to hold in the poop more when they are away from home than when they are at home. The home bathroom is familiar. The mother is at home to help wipe or with other aspects of the process. Away from home the bathroom might not be familiar and there is a difference in trust with non-mother caregivers. About seventy-five percent of school age children will not poop at school and wait until they get home. This process starts in daycare, pre-school, and kindergarten.

Third, once a child starts to leave home they learn to drink less away from home. They drink less so they don't have to use the bathroom as often. Pre-school children continue to drink liberally but by kindergarten the children learn to drink less. Drinking less makes the poop harder.

The slow methodical deterioration in bowel health from toilet training through to the elementary years is responsible for secondary onset day and night wetting. In children with secondary onset day and night wetting, there are months or years of dryness by day or by night before wetting intervenes.

The Influence of a New Sibling

Many parents and doctors blame "regression" of toilet training on the birth of a new sibling. When I was a young paediatrician, the conventional wisdom for this observation was sibling rivalry. According to this concept, the older child resented the attention conferred on the new baby and responded by wetting or pooping in their clothes. This is a myth. This does not happen.

I don't prefer the term "regression." I prefer to describe the situation as a "change" in bathroom behaviour. What changes is bowel health. Bowel health changes because the home environment changes with the delivery of a new sibling and bathroom behaviour in a toddler requires a lot of support from the parents.

The home environment changes radically with the birth of a new sibling. Pregnancy, labor, and delivery confer challenges on the mother. Most are tired, especially in the last trimester. Some continue to work outside the home. Some have a spouse who is supportive. Work and spousal support influences how tired a pregnant mother might be. Then the new baby is delivered. The sleep routine of the mother gets much worse and the mother is more tired. Mothers are obliged to carry on with the care necessary for the older siblings, the spouse, and the home, as well as for the new baby. Realistically something has to give. There are only so many hours in a day and the mother only has so much energy. Mothers are encouraged to allow about two years between each child. This allows the mother to recover and the baby to grow into a toddler before the next child arrives. With this spacing, the new baby arrives when the older child is walking, starting to separate from the mother, and beginning the exciting exploration of the home environment. The attention of the mother is appropriately directed at the new baby who is completely helpless and the mother spends less time with the older sibling. There is less focus on bathroom attendance and the bowel health of the older child changes. When bathroom behaviour of an older sibling changes after the birth of a new baby, this has nothing to do with sibling rivalry. This has everything to do with the limited ability of any mother to pay perfect attention to all the important maternal responsibilities in a home. In my experience, when the bathroom behaviour of an older sibling changes, a careful history usually reveals the child had some bowel and bladder control challenges in the year prior to the birth of the baby.

Many parents presume that once "toilet trained" a child will carry on independently and all will be well. For some children this happens. However, many children require ongoing support and encouragement to sustain good bathroom behaviour. Parents need to provide the structure for success with toilet training for as long as necessary. Less mature and busier children require more ongoing support during the pre-school years.

Two Basic Toilet Training Pre-requisites

The two basic pre-requisites that need to be in place for success with toilet training are good bowel health and average frontal lobe maturity for age.

1. Make sure the bowel health is bladder-friendly before toilet training. Track the poops in your child for at least a month before you plan to start toilet training. Change the hydration and fibre in the diet sufficiently to insure a minimum of one poop a day. Make sure the poop looks softer than paste. Use a poop softener as necessary.

2. Make sure the frontal lobe maturity is average for age. This is often referred to as "readiness." This is often the extent of the advice from most pediatricians. However, without good bowel health this is not enough. Readiness is present when there are signs the child recognizes they are peeing in the daytime diaper. The child will usually pause an activity, change their facial expression, or touch the genital area.

Toilet Training Techniques

✓ Chose a time when there is not much going on. Be home bodies. Set aside at least a long weekend.

✓ Strive for consistency. Discuss this as parents beforehand. Make sure you are both on the same behavioural page.

✓ Explain the process to your child. Lots of parents purchase a children's book on potty training and go over this in the days and weeks before they start.

✓ Start with a floor potty and graduate to the adult toilet with an over-the-toilet seat and a footstool. Allow the child to pick out the potty.

✓ Let your child sit on the potty with their clothes on until this is comfortable. Then let your child sit naked on the potty.

✓ Encourage your child to drink more than a bladder capacity. Offer diluted juice to guarantee compliance.

Once your child has a full bladder there are two common strategies.

1. Take off the clothes and allow your child to run around naked. With this technique you presume the child will tell you when they need to pee. You take them to the potty and supervise posture.

2. Ask your child to sit on the floor potty about every thirty minutes until they pee.

✓ Reward your child when they pee in the potty. Make this a big deal. Offer a treat.

✓ Ignore wet clothes but ask your child to tell you when they wet. Reward the child for telling you they wet so they can be promptly changed. Teach your child to **Value Dryness**.

Neurobiology – Daytime Wetting

The symptoms of daytime wetting are only recognized after toilet training. A child might have frequency with small volume pees while still in the diaper, but modern diapers are very absorbent, and for most mothers a wet diaper is just a wet diaper. Occasionally a very fastidious mother who is driven to change the diaper as often as necessary to ensure the infant is comfortable reports frequency. For all practical purposes, the symptoms of voiding problems are usually only noticeable when the diaper is removed with toilet training.

The average age a child is toilet trained in North America is about 2.5 years. At this age the average bladder should hold about 200 ml. At this age the frontal lobes are not well developed but the pace of neural development is accelerating. Toddlers are in a rapid learning phase as they explore their environment. They learn to separate from their mother and independently explore the world. There are new things to investigate and learn every day.

At a very basic level the kidneys make urine, the muscles in the ureters squirt the urine into the bladder, and the bladder fills up. There are pressure receptors in the bladder that detect bladder filling. Once the bladder is "full" a signal is sent up the spinal cord to the voiding center and then to the frontal lobes. The desired decision in the frontal lobes is to stop the current activity and proceed to the bathroom where the child can empty the bladder into the toilet.

The frontal lobes are obliged to process all the sensory information in the environment. Information on what the child sees (visual cortex), hears (auditory cortex), smells (olfactory lobes), touches (pressure sensations from other parts of the body), and tastes are transmitted to the frontal lobes for processing. The frontal lobes continue to develop until the age of about twenty-five years.

The emotional state of the child is monitored by the frontal lobes. Information on the emotional state is transmitted to the frontal lobes from the limbic system. Past experience (memory) is transmitted to the frontal lobes from the hippocampus.

When the signal of a full bladder reaches the frontal lobes, it is inevitable there will be signals from other parts of the brain. The signals compete with each other for predominance. I'm thinking of the hilarious donkey scene in Shrek, played so brilliantly by Eddie Murphy. The donkey is jumping up and down among a crowd of people and he shouts, "Pick me. Pick me." Making a decision to pay attention to the bladder signal, to "Pick me," is difficult when the development of the frontal lobes is modest and when there are multiple signals arriving from various parts of the brain. One way to think about this is the frontal lobes need to simultaneously arbitrate multiple tasks. Most people realize the difficulties with multi-tasking.

Daytime Wetting Usually Resolves by Grade Three

About seventy-five percent of children who wet the bed have a history of daytime wetting. The other twenty-five percent are dry by day and only wet at night. The timelines for natural resolution of the day and night wetting are different.

Daytime wetting usually resolves slowly from toilet training through to about the age eight years when most children are in grade three. Over this time the frequency of episodes of daytime wetting decrease and the volume of urine in the clothes gets less. A very common pattern is daytime wetting enough to change clothes in pre-school and kindergarten. Wetting enough to change the clothes resolves by the end of grade one. However, Mom still smells urine on her child when they get home from school and this resolves in grade two. Over the next year Mom still sees minor drip stains in the underwear when she does the laundry and this improves in grade three. Thereafter, the child still has urgency and might still wet the bed, but the daytime wetting resolves. This pattern evolves without ANY professional intervention. I recollect the moment when this pattern dawned on me. This was a major epiphany. Mostly this means daytime wetting gets better without my help. Kind of humbling. This process speeds up when bowel health is bladder-friendly.

The evolution is faster in some children and slower in others. Some make the transition to more attentive voiding and dryness before kindergarten. Some still struggle with this past grade three. Frontal lobe function likely plays a role in how fast a child makes this transition.

Social Evolution of Bathroom Behaviour

I call the slow resolution of daytime wetting over time the Social Evolution of Bathroom Behaviour. There are two reasons that account for this resolution of daytime wetting. First, the child learns to be more attentive (frontal lobe function) to the signals of the need to pee. Second, the child learns to drink less away from home.

Children learn from their peers. They want to conform with their peers. They don't want to wet in front of their peers. So, they learn to pee more often and to drink less while at school. The learning is a frontal lobe function. The children learn to do this but are not usually cognitively able to explain why they pee more attentively or drink less. I tell the parents that for these children the Force is with them. As Yoda taught, they "just do."

When I take a history from a parent, I start with toilet training and ask questions about the first year after toilet training, which is usually the first pre-school year. Then I ask questions about the second pre-school year, then kindergarten, then grade one, and so on until I reach the current year the child is in school. I ask about the prevalence of holding postures, urgency, and daytime wetting in each year. This takes time and sometimes tests the memory of the mother but the information has value. When the pattern reveals the expected slow resolution in daytime wetting over time, this is evidence the child is doing their part to help solve the problem. This information reassures the parent and helps the parent accept the situation. I also ask each child how often they pee during a typical school day. When a child tells me they pee three or more times, this confirms they are trying their best to be attentive to the signals of a full bladder and to stay in control. This also helps reassure the parent their child is doing their part. Parents are often overwhelmed by daytime wetting in their child. Some are impatient for dryness. The patience of a parent improves when they understand the problem is getting better, that their child is doing their part, and that the wetness will resolve. This information helps the parents see the light at the end of the daytime wetting tunnel.

School Wetting Resolves Before Home Wetting

Daytime wetting is usually more common at home than at school. Daytime wetting resolves at school before it does at home. There are reasons why wetting is less common at school and reasons why wetting is more common at home.

Wetting is less common at school because the child is with their peer group at school. The child socializes their bathroom behaviour first within the all-important peer group. Another reason is that the child does not usually drink much while at school.

Wetting is more common at home because the child returns home thirsty and has the biggest drink of the day when they get in the door. The small bladder fills up quickly and catches the child by surprise. At home the child is more likely to participate in more compelling play activities such as video games, television, or other activities that might distract a child from the signals.

Why Does Daytime Wetting Happen?

Daytime wetting happens when something interferes with the ability of a child to pay attention to the signal of a full bladder, to stop an activity, and go to the bathroom.

There are four situations that limit the ability of a child to pay attention to the signal of a full bladder, stop an activity, and go to the bathroom.

1. Bathroom access is a problem.
2. Child would rather play than pee and over time the child loses touch with the signals of a full bladder.

3. Child has a learning problem that affects frontal lobe function and interferes with the ability to process the signal of a full bladder.

4. Child has an emotional state that interferes with the ability to process the signal of a full bladder.

Bathroom Access

Lots of children wet when there is no bathroom nearby. They might be in a car or bus. They might be at a playground. Isolated wetting against a background of dryness is commonly due to a bathroom access problem.

Teachers often impose rules about when and how often a child can leave class to pee. These misguided rules oblige a child to hold the pee for the next authorized time to leave class. In a child with a small bladder that is up against a Poop Wall, this doesn't work. Some children are "rule followers," and this increases the risk for wetting at school when the rules are restrictive.

Sometimes an adult caregiver limits access. An impatient parent might not want to stop for a bathroom break on a road trip.

Child has a personality that would rather play than pee and over time the child loses touch with the signals of a full bladder

Personality plays a role in this decision. Some children are more inclined to pay prompt attention to the signals. I call these children **Attentive Voiders**. About twenty-five percent of the children who attend my clinic are Attentive Voiders. From toilet training they make the "hard decision" to stop their play activity and to attend in the bathroom and pee in the toilet. Perhaps they do not like the feeling of an overfull bladder. Perhaps they cannot accept the idea of wet clothes (loss of control). Mothers often score their Attentive Voider child higher on a perfectionist scale. I call this a personality trait, but this is still a cognitive frontal lobe decision. These children do not wet by day but they do drive their parents crazy peeing so often.

The other seventy-five percent of the children who attend my clinic are Less-Attentive Voiders. These children would rather play than pee. This makes perfect sense to a young child. These children suffer daytime wetting because they are not able to make the "hard decision" to stop a compelling play activity and go to the bathroom. The frontal lobes are where "hard decisions" are made. "Hard decisions" are decisions to do the "right thing." The "right thing" for a parent is for the child to go to the bathroom. The "right thing" for the child is to continue to play.

During compelling play, the frontal lobe of the child receives the signal of the need to pee. At the same time, the signal of the desire to continue the compelling play is also received by the frontal lobe. The child tries to respond to both signals by continuing to play but holding the pee in the bladder. The bladder pressure slowly but surely increases. There are limits to how long a child can hold the pee when the bladder is up against the Poop Wall. The daytime wetting happens because the compelling play signals processed in the developing frontal lobes take precedence over the stop and go pee signals. Remember the Shrek analogy.

Once a child starts to hold the pee past full during compelling play, they start to do this more and more. The early signals of a full bladder fade away much like background noise. Then the signals of an overfull bladder fade away, then the signals of a very overfull bladder fade away, and finally for some children, they are only aware of the need to pee when the urine starts to leak out into their clothes.

Some play activities are more compelling than others. Whether an activity is sufficiently compelling varies with the child. The more common compelling activities are video games, computer time, television, and play dates. For an occasional child reading is sufficiently compelling.

Video games are especially compelling. Wetting during video games is so common that jargon evolved to describe the episodes (Wii Wee, PlayStation Piddle). Daytime wetting during a video game was more common in the era when the games did not have a "pause" button. Playing video games might be addictive for some children. If this is the case, the decision to interrupt the video game and to pee is predictably very difficult. If a child is addicted to video game play, like every addiction, this is not something the child can control.

Child has a learning problem that affects frontal lobe function and interferes with processing the signal of a full bladder

Attention Deficit Hyperactivity Disorder (ADHD)

About twenty-five percent of children who attend my clinic have ADHD. The prevalence of ADHD in the general population is about five to ten percent. This implies that daytime and night wetting is more common in children with ADHD. My research published in 1997 was the first controlled study to establish this relationship. The relationship had been recognized by the specialists who treated children with ADHD for several decades prior to my study. One of these specialists was Dr. H. P. Jackson, who I worked with in South Carolina. Dr. Jackson and I discussed our observations on this association over a many lunches. Eventually we decided to do a controlled study. Our control group included children from the general pediatric clinic. The results published in 1997 show that at six years of age there is a significant increase in daytime wetting and bedwetting in children with ADHD. Daytime wetting is 4.5 times and bedwetting 2.6 times more common than in the control children. ADHD is the most common learning problem with impairment in the ability of the frontal lobes to process signals of the need to pee.

Autism

About eight percent of the children who attend my clinic have autism. Since the expected prevalence in childhood is 1.5 percent, this confirms day and night wetting is more common in children with autism. Frontal lobe problems with executive decisions and emotional regulation are present in some children with autism.

Children with autism have unique personal ways of problem solving. They often have practical solutions to problems other children would not come up with. I've learned to listen to these children.

Low blood sugar

Most mothers recognize that emotional lability in their child is triggered by low blood sugar. Cranky children need calories. Brain function is linked to glucose availability. Crankiness is a clue that frontal lobe function is impaired. If a busy child is running around burning off calories and the mother does not keep up the caloric intake, the blood sugar can fall and this impairs frontal lobe function. Daytime wetting is more common in children who skip meals or go long periods between eating.

Tiredness
Most mothers recognize that emotional lability in their child is triggered by tiredness. Cranky children need a nap. The crankiness is a clue that frontal lobe function is impaired. If a child is overtired, this impairs frontal lobe function. In pre-school children daytime wetting is more common in the afternoon just before nap time.

Abnormalities in the frontal lobe
Anything that damages the frontal lobes in a child either during the perinatal period or after birth might affect the ability to process the signal of a full bladder. Some of the more common causes include children with cerebral palsy due to perinatal asphyxia and children with Fetal Alcohol Syndrome. Children with global developmental delay or with intellectual disability likely have processing issues in their frontal lobes.

Child has an emotional state that interferes with processing the signal of a full bladder

Emotion routinely plays a role. An acutely stressful or exciting situation involves lots of signals from the limbic system to the frontal lobes. Acute stress in a child who is an Attentive Voider results in the need to pee more frequently with a smaller volume than usual. In a child who is not an Attentive Voider, the acute stress increases the risk of daytime wetting. Chronic emotional disorders such as anxiety and depression play a role in a similar fashion.

Many parents experiment with discipline when their child wets during the day. They mistakenly believe the child has a choice. They judge their child. They believe the child made a poor choice and deserves discipline. This is more common with poop accidents than with pee accidents. Another word for discipline is punishment. Yet another potential word is abuse. The spectrum of discipline can range from exasperation to emotional and physical abuse.

Imagine you are a toddler or pre-school child who wets by day. You have no ability to control the wetting because you have lost touch with the signals of a full bladder. Every time you wet your clothes the adults in the room get upset. There is a spectrum of upset. Perhaps the adult sighs. Perhaps their facial expression and body language is negative. Maybe they tell the child he or she is bad. Maybe the adult gets mad. Maybe the adult shames the child. Maybe the adult spanks the child. Regardless of the response by the adult, in all these situations the child feels bad. The child feels guilty. The child feels shame. When this happens on a regular basis the self-esteem of the child suffers. Eventually the relationship between the child and the adult suffers. Trust is lost. Thereafter every time the signal of a full bladder reaches the frontal lobes the memory of the shame, the guilt, and the punishment also reaches the frontal lobes. The emotions invoked with past episodes (anxiety, depression, anger) also reach the frontal lobes. Since the child does not have control because they have lost touch with the signals of a full bladder, the memories and the emotions that compete with the signal of a full bladder further limit the ability of the child to respond to the signal of a full bladder, and this makes the problem worse. As one wise Mom told me, nothing good comes from the "Blame Game."

Parents sometimes come to my clinic to seek approval to punish their child. Sometimes one parent believes in corporal punishment, sometimes both parents support this terrible practice. Mostly these parents are conflicted. They punish their child and feel bad because they know this is wrong. They know it isn't working. But in the absence of an alternative strategy, they ask for my approval to punish. I've learned to let these parents down softly. I explain the child has lost touch with the signals, that the child is not in control, that the child is not lying or naughty, and therefore the wetting is not the fault of the child. Many mothers start to cry when they realize this.

Some parents want my approval to judge their spouse who has a different response to the wetting. A mother might express her concern over the tough discipline meted out by her husband.

I always provide a written report of the discussion and recommendations to the parents. I write down that the child is not at fault and there is no role for punishment. I instruct the mother to provide the document for the father to read. I want the advice and recommendation to come directly from me through the written words, rather than from the mother.

When the mother and father separate or divorce and there is shared custody, and especially when the parental separation was acrimonious, one or both parents might seek to blame the other for day or night wetting. In some situations, this becomes part of a contentious court settlement. The child is the innocent victim in these between-parent conflicts. My role is to insure both homes communicate and apply the management principles in a consistent pattern. Often easier said than done.

Memory plays a role. The hippocampus and other parts of the limbic system store memory information. Sometimes memory improves frontal lobe function and sometimes memory complicates frontal lobe function.

Memory improves frontal lobe function in some children. When I dig down into the past history in a child who is an especially Attentive Voider, sometimes there is a history of an early embarrassing wetting episode, typically when bathroom access was a problem for the child. Often this is the only time a child had an embarrassing wetting episode. Many times, the child remembers and the mother doesn't! The memory of this especially embarrassing episode lingers sufficiently to make the child more attentive to early bladder signals. These children learn strategies to stay dry. They learn where all the bathrooms are in a school or shopping mall. They plan their day to insure good bathroom access. This planning is a frontal lobe function. These children sometimes panic when they need to pee and bathroom access is limited such as during car rides.

Memory complicates frontal lobe function in some children. This is common in children who are shamed or punished for daytime wetting. Punishment is never appropriate. The spectrum of punishment extends from mild looks of exasperation to physical abuse. The memories of the punishment are stored in the hippocampus and other parts of the limbic system. Connections from limbic system to the frontal lobes activate an emotion (shame, guilt, pain, anxiety). The emotion signals compete with the signal to stop an activity and go pee.

Two Basic Patterns of Daytime Wetting

Hold, Run, and Wet
The child holds the pee past full, runs to pee at the last minute, and wets before they reach the bathroom. With this pattern the parent can see the tell-tale holding postures that confirm the bladder is full.

Just Wet
In the other basic pattern of wetting the child wets without any discernable change in posture. The child suddenly just empties the bladder into their clothes. The parent does not see any of the tell-tale signs of holding. One moment the child is dry. The next moment the child is wet.

Hold, Run, and Wet

This is the most common of the basic patterns. The child holds the pee past full, runs to pee, and wets before they reach the bathroom. The parent can see the tell-tale holding postures that confirm the bladder is full.

The spectrum of holding postures is wide. At one end of the spectrum is the classic pee-pee dance. The child bounces from one foot to the other. Earlier in the spectrum there is an increase in motor activity in the legs. The motor activity in the legs might reflect learned changes in response to tension of the pelvic floor muscles. In my office the child sits across from me in a chair. As soon as the child sits forward or suddenly stands up, this means they need to pee.

Some parents know by a change in facial expression before any motor activity in the legs. Some parents know by a change in the emotional state. In my office, the children start to get busier, to distract their mother more often, to drop crayons or pencils. When I see these behaviours I know the child has a full bladder.

In children who hold the pee past full their ability to sense the early signals of fullness eventually fade away much like background noise. This analogy helps parents to understand what is happening. The neurological mechanism for the disappearance of background noise is called accommodation. The sound is still present in the environment. The auditory cortex still records the noise but the frontal lobes do not make the individual aware of the noise. This is convenient so the individual is not distracted by the noise and can focus cognition on something else. The same process occurs with smells. When a person walks into a home with a smell (good or bad) the smell is initially strong but then disappears. The smell is still registered in the olfactory lobes but the frontal lobes make the smell disappear. The frontal lobes can accommodate any sensory signal (vision, hearing, smell, taste, and touch). The pressure signals in the bladder fall under the touch category.

When the signals fade away, this is convenient for the child because this allows the child to continue to focus on their preferred activity. The signals of bladder fullness can be suppressed so efficiently by the frontal lobes that the child can be posturing, seconds away from wetting, or even in the process of wetting, and not realize the bladder is full.

When a parent notes typical holding postures in their child, they usually ask the child to pee. They are sometimes perplexed when their child responds they don't need to pee. This denial is evidence of how effectively the frontal lobes can suppress the pressure signals in the bladder. I make a point to tell the parents that the child is not lying. Rather, the child has lost touch with the signals. The child does not have control over this process. I explain the background noise analogy. When the child denies they need to pee notwithstanding obvious holding postures, this can lead to a confrontation between the parent and child. Confrontations do not help. Once the child is embroiled in the confrontation, the emotion signals from the limbic system likely preclude any possibility the child will recognize the signal of the need to pee. When a child denies they need to pee in this situation, some parents judge their child. Some parents tell me their child is stubborn or will-full. Other parents tell me the child is lying. Some describe the episode as a "control" situation. Some punish their child. **I explain that losing touch with the signal of a full bladder is not the fault of the child. The child does not have control. There is no role for punishment.**

Most parents try to explain the situation to their child and expect the child to understand. Logic and reason is often not an effective way to influence the behavior of a pre-school or early elementary school aged child.

One mother offered a unique solution to help her kindergarten-aged child understand he had lost touch with the signals. The mother had patiently tried many times to explain to her son that when she sees the holding postures he needs to stop what he is doing and go pee to avoid a wetting episode. The explanations fell on deaf ears. This ingenious mother set up a video camera and gave her son some juice to drink. Juice is an uncommon treat in the home and the boy rapidly drank a whole cup. The mother waited patiently while the boy played with Lego. She turned the camera on and recorded quiet play and then the transition to motor activity in the legs. Mom asked her son to go to the bathroom when she saw the pee-pee dance. She also recorded her voice with a description of what she saw. She recorded her son's denial of the need to pee. The camera continued to record the next few minutes as the posturing increased, and the final frames recorded the boy urgently running to the bathroom holding his penis. Later, once optimally rested and fed, and therefore receptive to learning, Mom showed him the video. The boy learned to be more attentive to the signals and the wetting decreased. The frontal lobes in this boy were developed enough to be receptive to this learning experience.

A mother of a kindergarten-aged girl told me her daughter wet more often when her little brother was in the same room. The girl was protective about her toys. The little brother often tried to take them when she wasn't looking. When the mother noted posturing in the daughter and the little brother was around, the mother learned to remind the girl to pee and also to promise to guard the toys.

Some children are able to problem solve the process more than others. One mother related that her 6-year-old boy regularly held his pee past full while playing. She reminded him when she saw the posturing. When he doesn't stop the play activity and proceed to the bathroom, she ups the stakes. The mother tells her son she is going to use the solitary bathroom in the home. With this new information the boy stops the play activity and goes to the bathroom. In a similar fashion a father told his son that he would lock the bathroom doors if he doesn't stop the play and go pee.

Not every child denies they need to pee while posturing. Many children accept the advice of their parent and attend the bathroom. Some parents report their child seems to "think" about the request and then agree. I see this in my office all the time. I see the posturing and ask the child to pee. Some deny. However, some pause their activity, look up as if they are thinking, then agree. The ones who are thinking are accessing their frontal lobes. When a child "looks up," this is a nifty body language metaphor that depicts access to the frontal lobes.

Voiding at Transition Times

Children who are not Attentive Voiders need to be reminded to pee to minimize daytime wetting. At home the child should be encouraged to void at the common transition times. Transition times are always before something. Before meals, before going outside to play, before a play date, before watching television, before starting a video game, and before they get in the car. Transition times are also when you wake up and before bed. There are enough common transition times in a home day to keep a child dry, but this is a lot of work for the parent. When a parent sees holding postures in their child, this implies the parent missed an opportunity to remind the child to pee at an earlier transition time. Not every parent is up for working on transition time voiding. Some accept the wetting and carry on. I have a lot of respect for the parents who can make this work. Takes the right parent and the right child working together. At follow up visits I inquire about how often a child wets by day and the circumstances. The parents who make transition time work often comment, "He's much better. When he does wet, it's my fault. The wetting happens when I'm too busy to remind him." I want to high five these parents. I am proud of them. They have accepted their responsibility to structure voiding. I compliment these parents on their extraordinary efforts and empathy.

If a child is posturing during a compelling play activity the child will not usually cooperate to pee when reminded by the parent. The child has lost touch with the signals of bladder fullness and does not realize they need to pee. The parent knows but the child doesn't know. What the child does know is they want to keep playing. This setting is often the trigger for a confrontation. Rather than risk a confrontation in this setting I recommend the parent "finesse" a transition. This requires finding a suitable distraction that will interrupt the compelling play. Perhaps the mother can suggest a healthy treat the child enjoys. "Bobbie would you like one the oatmeal cookies mommy baked?" On the way to the kitchen, no longer engrossed in the compelling play, the mother reminds the child to pee in the bathroom. Everyone wins. Bobby gets a treat. Mom finesses cooperation. Bobby is dry. Best of all, there is no confrontation.

Transition time voiding makes good sense to the parent but not always to the child. Some children deny they need to pee when requested to pee at a common transition time. In some children the denial of the need to pee turns into a refusal to pee. Finessing the request is a challenge for some parents. Sometimes a confrontation develops. The confrontation develops because the parent believes the child is "stubborn" or "lying." The child is neither. If a child does not feel like they need to pee, the child presumes the bladder is empty, and the request by the parent does not make sense to the child. Before the age of eight or nine years, children do not understand the concept of a partially full bladder. For young children the bladder is either full or empty. One way of thinking about this is that the concept of a partially full bladder requires knowledge of the mathematical concept of "fractions." Another way of thinking about this is a partially full bladder is an "abstract" concept. Children don't learn about "fractions" until the middle years of elementary school and "abstract" concepts are sometimes not understood until middle school. I explain this to parents who end up in confrontations over voiding at transition times. Confrontations lead to emotional memories around voiding that interfere with the ability to pay attention to the early signals of bladder fullness. Confrontations can have a negative effect on the relationship between the child and parent. Confrontations are never helpful.

Many parents use a watch alarm to remind their child to pee more often. If you have a child who is a rule follower, a watch alarm might help.

Transition time voiding and watch alarms can minimize wetting but neither strategy teaches a child to respond to the early signals of fullness. This is something the child will do on their own once they start to socialize with their peers at school. Their peers will be mostly dry and peer-dryness sets the social standard for the child to emulate.

Identifying the signal of a full bladder is a greater challenge for some children. I review a variety of strategies to help these children. The goal is for them to learn to "listen to their body." One strategy is to increase the pressure on the bladder so they can appreciate the signal. Standing increases the pressure. Many children do not feel full while in the car on the way to my clinic but realize they need to pee as soon as they get out of the car and walk into the clinic. When I see body language clues that suggest a child has a full bladder, I ask the child if they need to pee and they often respond, "No." Then I ask the child to stand and think about the bladder. When they stand some realize they need to pee. Or, I ask the child to stand and walk and think about the bladder. Another strategy is to remove external stimuli. I ask the child to stand and close their eyes and think about the bladder. Or stand, walk out of the room (leave a busy environment and find a quiet place), and think about the bladder. I tell the children these techniques are a "Bladder Scan." These are attempts to help the child recognize the signal of a full bladder even when they do not think the bladder is full. When I ask a child whether they need to pee, a common answer is "Kinda." I explain that "kinda" is the early signal of the need to pee and suggest that the child learn to pee when they feel "kinda" full.

Getting back in touch with the earlier signals of bladder fullness takes time and practice. Getting back in touch is much faster once the bowel health is "bladder-friendly." Once the bladder is surrounded by soft poop, the bladder can push the poop out of the way. This gives the child more time to learn to pay attention to the signal of fullness.

Role of the teacher

Teachers specify a variety of bathroom rules. The rules vary teacher to teacher and not generally school to school. About ten years ago I did a survey of the school bathroom rules in the children who attended my clinic. I asked one hundred and twenty-five consecutive children in grades one to three to tell me about the rules in their school. I was flabbergasted by what I learned.

A common rule is to limit the number of times a child can attend the bathroom during the school day. Commonly the bathroom breaks are limited to two during the day. This doesn't work for children with a smaller bladder. Limiting bathroom breaks guarantees a child will drink less.

Another common rule is to request the child wait until the next convenient break (snack, recess, lunch). This is wrong because the teacher is encouraging (teaching) a child to hold the pee past full. Most of the children don't need any practice!

There are a variety of different hand signals and sign out procedures. A child might need to place something on their desk when they leave class. One teacher used a toy bathroom plunger. LOL. A child might be asked to write their name on a clip board or a white board. Some teachers rely on hand signals.

Some children are embarrassed to use a hand signal, to follow a sign out procedure, or to otherwise ask to pee. These requests in front of peers are intimidating for some children and embarrassing for others. A child does not need to ask to pee at home. Parents don't restrict bathroom access at home. Teachers shouldn't restrict access at school.

The rule I teach is that a child should **ALWAYS leave class to pee** and never be wait for a break. Teachers should allow easy access to the bathroom as often as necessary. Parents need to communicate these rules to the teacher. I write lots of notes to teachers to request their help.

Many teachers presume that some children ask to leave class to pee because they are bored or want to escape class work. The majority of children who ask to leave class need to pee. Teachers should always believe the child.

The information in my survey that really offended me is that some teachers punish children for going to the bathroom. In my survey four percent of the teachers punished children for peeing too often! The punishments ranged from limiting privileges, to extra classroom work, to after school detentions. I consider this a form of child abuse.

Don't teach a child to hold the pee past full

Half a century ago someone popularized the idea that a bladder gets bigger if you practice holding the pee past full. This is sometimes referred to as "bladder-retention-training." There is no truth to his myth but some physicians still recommend hold the pee exercises. This doesn't work and leads to all the negative consequences noted above. These children don't need practice holding the pee past full, most are already holding their pee way too much on their own!

Teach Your Child to Value Dryness

Many parents are concerned when their child continues to play in wet clothes. This is common when daytime wetting is daily. Toddlers are more likely to play in wet clothes than elementary-aged children. The parents often report the child "cannot feel" the wetness. The parents worry this implies a nerve problem. There is no nerve problem. The child is not lying. The child has accommodated to the sensation of wetness.

Some parents get upset when their child continues to play in wet clothes and even more upset when the child denies they are wet. Confrontations are more common when parents get upset. Confrontation never helps. I teach the parents that this is not the fault of the child.

A child who continues to play in wet clothes needs to learn to **Value Dryness**. The more they play in wet clothes, the more they will accommodate to wet clothes, and the more they will continue to play in wet clothes. The parent needs to change this pattern. The child needs to be experience dryness for longer and longer periods of time. They need to learn that dryness has a value.

I recommend a specific behavioural intervention for a child to learn to value dryness. First, the parent needs to reassure the child they will not be punished for wetting. The parent needs to stop the Blame Game. Second, the parent needs to explain to the child that dryness is important. The rational might be lost on young children but I recommend parents give the child the benefit of the doubt. Dryness is a social goal. The mother might say, "Mommy is dry and she wants you to be dry." Mothers need to explain that dryness is important to prevent rashes or discomfort in the genital area. Third, the mother needs to tell the child that every time the child wets and tells the mother right away the mother will reward the child with a treat. This might take weeks of practice, but over time, this Value Dryness practice helps the child learn to stay dry longer. Learning to Value Dryness in isolation isn't enough. The mother must also work on bowel health and help the child to be more attentive to the early bladder signals.

Some parents have difficulty accepting my Value Dryness recommendations. They believe that rewarding a child when they tell you they wet is the same as rewarding a child for wetting. This is not the case. If the recommendations are applied consistently and with empathy, the child will learn to Value Dryness. Avoiding the Blame Game is very important.

Negative Consequences of Holding the Pee Past Full
Holding the pee past full has negative consequences apart from the risk of daytime wetting. There are physical, cognitive, and emotional consequences.

Physical Consequences of Holding the Pee Past Full
Chronically holding the pee past full is accomplished by tension in the pelvic floor muscles. I regularly see spontaneous pelvic floor muscle contractions when I do a pelvic ultrasound. This implies the pelvic floor muscles are tense. Tension in the pelvic floor muscles can interfere with bladder and bowel emptying.

The physical consequence of an overfull bladder is thickening of the bladder wall. The bladder wall is a muscle and the muscle cells get bigger under pressure. If a child is an Attentive Voider, the bladder wall thickness measured in an empty bladder (defined as less than 5 ml of urine) is less then 3 mm. In a child who holds the pee past full, the bladder wall is thicker and the diameter is greater than 3 mm. I regularly see bladder walls as thick as 4 to 5 mm in children who chronically hold the pee past full over a period of years. The thickest bladder wall I've measured in a child is 9 mm.

The thickness of the bladder wall is related to the number of years since toilet training that the child has held the urine past full, to how frequently the child holds the urine past full, and to the presence of specific patterns of holding behaviour adopted by the child.

Most children who hold the pee past full do so from toilet training but some learn to do this later after toilet training as the bowel health worsens and the bladder capacity decreases. About a quarter of the children who hold the urine past full start this during kindergarten or grade one. The bladder wall thickness is related to the duration in years that the child has held the urine past full.

Some children hold the urine past full away while at school, some while at home, and some in both situations. Some hold the urine past full intermittently and others hold the urine past full routinely. Intermittent patterns at school vary depending on bathroom access and school activities. Intermittent patterns at home very depending on play activities. Children who routinely hold the pee past full in both settings have thicker bladder walls than children who only hold the pee past full in one of the settings or only intermittently.

Some children do not pee at school. The most common reason for not peeing at school is that the child does not drink anything while away from home. However, a smaller group of children do not pee at school for other reasons. There are three common reasons why a child does not pee at school. Some children find school bathrooms offensive from a hygiene perspective. Some children experienced bullying in a school bathroom. Some children are determined not to miss out on classwork or social activities. Other less common reasons for not peeing at school include fear of bathroom ghosts (this was common after the Harry Potter book with Moaning Myrtle was released) and fear of being trapped in a school bathroom during a fire alarm drill, which for young child can be a terrifying experience with strong negative memories that linger.

Some of the children who will not pee at school learn behaviours to help them hold the urine past full. From elementary and especially from middle to late elementary some of these children are able to describe the behaviours they employ to hold the pee past full. Some children explain how they tense up their pelvic floor muscles to keep the pee in. They tell me they squeeze their thighs together, scrunch up their bum cheeks, and "suck the pee back in." Some hold the pee in under such high pressure they develop pain in the bladder (suprapubic or lower abdominal pain). Some even develop pain in the kidney (low back, flank, or side pain). Some children wait for these body language clues to develop before they finally leave class to pee! The bladder wall thickness in these children is routinely over 5 mm.

Some children acknowledge they routinely let a small amount of pee out of the bladder to reduce the pressure and to allow them time to either get to the bathroom or to reach the end of the school day. These children let off only a little pee and the pressure in the bladder stays chronically high. The muscle gets thicker and the bladder wall thickness measurement is usually over 5 mm.

Cognitive Consequences of Holding the Pee Past Full

The cognitive consequence of an overfull bladder is an inability to concentrate on the immediate task (classroom or play). Most parents can recollect personal situations in a meeting or lecture after drinking too much coffee or tea. They feel the need to pee but don't want to interrupt the meeting or speaker. They try to hold their pee and wait for the break. Most realize they are not able to concentrate in this situation. In school, when a teacher asks a child to wait to pee, the teacher, unwittingly, has compromised learning.

Emotional Consequences of Holding the Pee Past Full

The child's emotional state can change when they hold the pee. This might be expressed with emotional lability or anger. Changes in mood are likely more common with an overfull bladder than commonly recognized. I recommend parents look for these patterns and ask their child to void when they observe a sudden change in mood.

One mother told me she could tell when her elementary-aged son had to pee because he became aggressive to his younger brother. He pestered him. Once the mother recognized this pattern, she asked the older brother to pee every time he started to pester the younger brother.

One toddler in my office was aggressive playing with a toy truck on the floor. As the bladder filled past full the boy started to drive the truck into the chair, exam table, or wall. I asked the boy to pee and his aggressive behaviour settled. The bladder filled up again and the aggressive behaviour resumed. After he peed, he settled. I triggered this behaviour three times in a row so the mother could appreciate the pattern. She didn't believe me until the third episode.

Just Wet

The other basic pattern of wetting in a child is when the child wets without any discernable change in posture. The child suddenly empties the bladder into their clothes. The parent does not see any of the tell-tale signs of holding. One moment the child is dry. The next moment the child is wet.

One day my assistant overheard a six-year-old girl talking to a four-year-old girl in the play area of my reception room. The little girl was posturing. The big girl offered her advice. "Just wet your clothes. I do it all the time." Taken literally this implies the six-year-old makes a frontal lobe decision to empty her bladder and not to attend the bathroom to void in the toilet. Until this episode, I presumed all children Hold and Run and Wet. This episode taught me to look for the Just Wet pattern.

There are two common factors associated with the Just Wet pattern. There is a very small bladder capacity and the child is younger.

The bladder capacity in children who Just Wet is usually less than twenty-five percent of average. With a very small bladder capacity the child needs to void very frequently. My sense is there is a limit to how often a child will void before they give up and Just Wet.

The age of the child likely reflects frontal lobe maturity. The Just Wet pattern is most common in the months immediately after toilet training and often extends through the first year or two. Toddlers with a very small bladder find it very easy to carry on with the pre-toilet training pattern. They Just Wet, much as they did when they were in a diaper.

The table below compares outcome scenarios for Hold, Run, and Wet (HRW) and Just Wet (JW) based on bladder size and age (frontal lobe maturity). Older (higher frontal lobe maturity) children with larger bladder sizes are dry. Younger (lower frontal lobe maturity) children with the smallest bladder size Just Wet. Hold, Run, and Wet gets more common as the bladder gets bigger and the age increases (frontal lobe maturity improves).

Bladder size compared to average for age	Frontal Lobe Maturity for age - High	Frontal Lobe Maturity for age - Average	Frontal Lobe Maturity for age - Low
75%	Dry No Urgency	Dry Urgency	HRW
50%	Dry Urgency	HRW	JW
25%	HRW	JW	JW

The Just Wet pattern in a child with a very small bladder who has just been toilet trained makes sense. Before toilet training, the child Just Wet into the diaper. The child continues to do what they know. Once a child starts to leave home for school in kindergarten and grade one, the Just Wet pattern evolves into a Hold, Run, and Wet pattern. This happens because the child is with their peer group and wants to emulate peer-group behaviour. The bladder is still smaller than average, perhaps even smaller because the bowel health usually gets worse from toilet training to grade one. The transition to Hold, Run, and Wet is therefore likely a function of frontal lobe development.

When the pattern reveals the expected slow transition from Just Wet to Hold, Run, and Wet, this implies the child is doing their part to help solve the problem. I point this out to the parent. This information reassures the parent and helps the parent accept the situation. Parents are often overwhelmed by daytime wetting in their child. Some are impatient for dryness. The patience of a parent improves when they understand the problem is getting better, that their child is doing their part.

Achieving bladder-friendly bowel health will speed up the transition from Just Wet to Hold, Run, and Wet.

The bladder wall thickness in children who Just Wet is different than the bladder wall thickness in children who Hold, Run, and Wet. The bladder wall thickness in the children who Just Wet is normal and less than 3 mm. The bladder wall thickness in children who Hold, Run, and Wet is thicker than normal and usually in the range of 3 to 5 mm.

The Just Wet pattern is more common in children on the Autism spectrum. These children often make decisions that are logical and sensible from their unique perspective. They don't see any reason not to continue with their preferred activity. Neither do they see any reason to suffer the uncomfortable consequences of holding the pee past full. They "Just Wet" and continue this pattern until older than children who do not have autism and who "Just Wet." I recollect an eleven-year old girl with autism who "Just Wet" when she was engrossed in reading. The Just Wet pattern is uncommon after kindergarten. When I see an elementary aged child who still has the "Just Wet" pattern, I start to consider whether the child is on the Autism spectrum.

Don't Go Back into Diapers
When wetting is daily with multiple changes of clothes each day, some parents put their child back in a diaper. This is not a good idea. This allows the child to Just Wet into the diaper and to resume the pre-toilet training pattern. Once back in the diaper, there is no need for the frontal lobes to pay attention to the signals of a full bladder.

Daytime wetting is a trigger for social embarrassment and bullying at school
Daytime wetting is a bigger social issue than bedwetting because the wetting is public and in the presence of peers. Most parents are keen to solve the daytime wetting problem because they don't want their child to be shamed at school. This is a real concern and an important reason to help these children and their families.

During pre-school there are so many children who wet by day that this is not a concern. There are still about five to ten percent of children who wet by day in kindergarten. Shaming during the pre-school and early elementary years, when it does occur, is mostly done by the adult teachers and caregivers. By grade four classmates start to participate in shaming. This is the age when the prevalence of bullying at school starts to increase. Children with daytime wetting beyond grade four are at serious risk for shaming and bullying at school. These children often do not appreciate their risk. The mother can smell the child when they get home from school. The mother worries for the child because the mother knows if she can smell the child, others can too. However, the child cannot smell the urine. This smell disappears, is accommodated by the brain of the child, much as people with body odour and bad breath cannot appreciate how bad they smell to others. I make this clear to children from grade three on so they can do their part to pee more attentively and minimize their risk for embarrassment.

Summary of Treatment of Daytime Wetting

1. Make sure there is no underlying physical problem.

2. Look for bladder infection (especially in girls) and treat as necessary.

3. Explain that the wetting is because the bladder is smaller due to poop pressure.

4. Explain that how a child pays attention to bladder signals plays an important role.

5. Achieve bladder-friendly bowel health

6. Ensure bathroom access is good at school and otherwise while away from home.

7. Stop the Blame Game. Make sure all the adult caregivers understand the wetting is not the fault of the child. The child has lost touch with the signals. Do not judge, shame, or otherwise punish the child. Don't add an emotional component to the process since this will complicate the ability of the child to make a decision to stop an activity and go pee.

8. Help your child get back in touch with the early bladder signals. Teach your child to void at the common transition times. Teach your child to leave class to pee and never wait for a break. Teach your child how to listen to their body and do a "bladder scan."

9. Teach your child to Value Dryness.

10. Don't go back into diapers.

11. Be patient. Daytime wetting usually slowly improves over time even without intervention.

Small Bladder Volume Syndromes with Day or Night Wetting

There are four small bladder volume syndromes

1. Frequency

2. Nocturia

3. Getting up from the supper table to pee

4. Sensation of wetness or the need to void again immediately after a routine void

Frequency

How often a child pees depends on the size of the bladder and the amount of pee the kidneys make. Since most of the children with frequency learn not to drink very much, the major factor is usually the size of the bladder.

One exception is when a child is offered juice or pop. Modern mothers limit these sweet drinks for health reasons but continue to offer these drinks as "treats." These sweet drinks are compelling and a child will often guzzle the entire drink in one big gulp. After a larger drink over a short period of time, the bladder fills up multiple times over the next hour and triggers frequency or an episode of wetting. In these settings, the small bladder is "exposed" by drinking more than usual.

The small bladder is almost always due to poop pressure at the bottom of the pelvis. Bladder infection should always be considered, especially in girls.

The Role of Personality in Voiding Frequency

About twenty-five percent of the children who attend my clinic are Attentive Voiders. These children routinely pee more often than their peers with a similar sized bladder. They do this because their personality (frontal lobes) is driven to routinely make the harder decision to stop an activity and go to the bathroom. Either they do not enjoy the sensation of an overfull bladder or the possibility of wetting is not something they are willing to entertain. Sometimes there is a memory (hippocampus) of a solitary emotionally traumatic wetting episode. After such an episode the child might have an exaggerated fear (amygdala) of wetting.

Attentive voiding is more common in children whose parents score them high on the perfectionist scale, in children who have obsessive compulsive traits, and in children with anxiety.

Children with these personality traits void more often than might be accounted for by the poop pressure on the bladder.

Nocturia

Nocturia means the child needs to wake up to pee. This is the nighttime equivalent of voiding frequently during the day. Nocturia almost always implies the bladder size is reduced below average for age. Less commonly, nocturia is because the kidneys make too much pee overnight. Diabetes mellitus and diabetes insipidus can cause overproduction of urine by day and by night and is a cause of nocturia.

If a child is dry at night and can wake to pee, the bladder size is more than fifty percent of average. In a child who wets the bed and who never wakes to pee, the bladder size is less than fifty percent of average. The difference is related to when the bladder fills up during the sleep cycle. A bladder capacity less than fifty percent implies multiple fillings overnight and the first filling early in the sleep cycle. A bladder capacity greater than fifty percent implies only one filling later in the sleep cycle. The prevalence of deep sleep is higher early in the sleep cycle and lower later in the sleep cycle. It is easier to wake up during the lighter stages of sleep.

About ten percent of grade one children commonly wake up to pee and are dry at night. A similar percent of grade one children wet the bed and do not wake up to pee. Both groups of children have smaller bladders due to poop pressure. Those who are dry and wake up to pee have bladders that fill up only once later in the sleep cycle. Those who are wet and don't wake up to pee have bladders that fill up multiple times including early in the sleep cycle when the deeper stages of sleep are more prevalent.

I have never had a child referred to my clinic with the concern that the child wakes to pee. A child who wakes to pee has a smaller bladder than average and this is invariably due to poop pressure but since the child is dry at night, the parents do not consider waking to pee a concern.

Getting up from the supper table to pee

Most of the children who attend my clinic get up from the supper table to pee at least a few times every week. Some parents presume this is a ruse to get away from the dinner table to avoid eating or to engage in play activity. This is a legitimate need to pee situation. The sequence of events that come together to cause this behaviour includes five steps.

1. The child arrives home from school dehydrated and has the biggest drink of the day with their after-school snack. Some children have a second drink between home time and supper time. The kidneys respond to the hydration and make pee which is delivered to the bladder.

2. The child did not poop after breakfast, after lunch, or after school. There is therefore lots of poop in the rectum and this poop is pressing on the bladder and the bladder size is compromised.

3. The child starts to eat dinner and this initiates the gastro-colic reflex. The muscles in the intestine contract to push the poop along and make room for the soon to arrive ingested food.

4. The gastrocolic reflex increases the pressure in the rectum and this increases the pressure in the bladder.

5. The child appropriately picks up on the signal of the need to pee and leaves the dinner table. This is really a signal of the need to pee and to poop and some children do poop at this time. Others hold the poop in and only pee.

Sensation of wetness or the sensation of the need to pee again immediately after a routine void

The first time I recognized this pattern of symptoms was about thirty years ago. In 1993 I reported four girls with what I then called Post-Micturition Dribble Syndrome.

The girls describe the sensation of urine coming out after a routine void. Sometimes they tell their mother they feel wet. Sometimes they tell their mother they need to pee again. Immediately after a routine pee, they return to sit on the toilet but either no urine or perhaps a drip comes out. The mothers look between the labia and are perplexed because the child reports urine is coming out, but the Mom does not see any dampness. The girls routinely wipe the genital area to mop up any drips. They go back and forth to the bathroom, sometimes as many as ten times! Some learn to stuff tissue in their underwear. Since 1993, I've seen several hundred girls with this symptom. They are often referred for "frequency" because they feel like they need to pee again and go back and forth into the bathroom so many times. I don't call this frequency. I call this the sensation of wetness or the sensation of the need to pee again immediately after a routine void.

The sensation is intermittent and not with every void. The sensation is more common after a larger void, such as a first morning pee. The sensation waxes and wanes and then slowly resolves, but this might take months or even years. Over time, the girl returns to the bathroom less and less often. Finally, I think they learn to ignore the sensation and otherwise carry on. The disappearance of the symptom is likely a frontal lobe function. Likely the symptom is accommodated by the frontal lobes. The frontal lobes make the symptom disappear.

I see this almost exclusively in girls usually in the pre-school, kindergarten or early elementary grades. There is never a story of real daytime wetting, holding postures or urgency. These girls are all Attentive Voiders, usually right from toilet training. They stop what they are doing and go pee without reminders from parents. There might be a problem with bedwetting but this is not consistently present. This symptom is very frustrating. Some of the girls get emotionally distraught and cry.

There is never infection in the urine. The children have a normal bladder wall thickness. They always empty the bladder totally. This is important to demonstrate and discuss with the parents who sometimes think the back-and-forth to the bathroom symptom implies the bladder did not empty.

The bowel health varies but is usually not terrible. They often miss a few days a week and have hard poop with a random pattern but constipation symptoms are uncommon.

The symptom is likely due to a bladder "after-contraction." An after-contraction is when the bladder muscle contracts again after a normal void. These girls learn to appreciate the sensation of a bladder contraction with a routine void. When these girls feel the same sensation with an after-contraction, they expect urine to come out but with an after-contraction there is no longer any urine in the bladder. When this first starts to happen, the girl does not know there is no urine in the bladder. All they know is that this sensation usually means urine will come out. The girl expects to be wet if she doesn't return to the toilet. So she goes back and forth into the bathroom.

There is a personality that is susceptible to this symptom. I suspect the sensation is experienced by lots of girls, but ignored by most. Girls with a particular personality cannot ignore the symptom, at least not at the onset. I call this the Princess and the Pea Syndrome. In this famous Hans Christian Anderson fairy tale, the girl feels a pea under twelve mattresses! Only a real princess could feel a pea, much as only these girls feel the bladder after-contraction. A surprising number of these girls arrive in my office with clothes and gear that has a Disney Princess theme! The parents usually score these children high on the perfectionist scale. The symptom is more common in children with anxiety disorder. Occasionally there is a past history of a solitary emotionally significant wetting episode in the pre-school years, usually in a setting with limited bathroom access. These girls often panic when they are in car and feel the need to pee because there is no bathroom nearby.

Poop pressure on the bladder might play a role. I wonder if the sensation is triggered by solid stool settling on the empty bladder as the girl stands up to pull up their underwear and pants. This fits with the symptom occurring more often after a larger bladder is emptied. When a large bladder empties there is a temporary "void" and solid stool might settle into this space and onto the bladder and trigger the after contraction. Softening the stool and working on a first AM poop routine reduces but does not eliminate the symptom. I teach that the problem is due to poop and personality, with an emphasis on the personality. This is an important teaching point because I cannot change the personality. I can change the poop.

I always explain the symptom thoroughly and reassure the mother that the problem, while very frustrating is not serious. I explain the symptom will eventually fade away. I tell the children to try to ignore the symptom. I make recommendations to soften up the stool and achieve a first morning poop pattern.

One of the few males I assessed with this problem was a 17 year-old boy with autism. He was non-verbal but his Mom was a great historian. He had a longstanding history of constipation that Mom usually kept under good control with a stool softener. The onset of the "after contraction" symptom coincided with an acute change in his bowel health with multiple missed days without a poop. The adolescent responded by sitting on the toilet for up to 20 minutes after a routine void. The mom reported an initial large and typical gush of urine but then little or nothing thereafter for the twenty minutes her son continued to sit. Mom reports that he was an Attentive Voider from the age of 7 years when Mom stopped the daytime diaper. He refused to leave the house without voiding.

Wetting with Laughter

1. Giggle Incontinence
2. Stress Incontinence

Giggle Incontinence

In Giggle Incontinence the bladder totally empties. The child is usually soaked. There is no pee in the bladder when the child goes to the bathroom immediately after the episode.

Giggle Incontinence is almost always in girls. The wetting occurs with "hearty" laughter, a real belly laugh. The wetting starts in pre-school or early elementary-aged girls and often, but not always resolves by adulthood. There is sometimes a family history in the mother or grandmother. Giggle Incontinence is embarrassing for the girl.

The wetting is due to sudden uncontrolled relaxation of the external sphincter, the muscle that wraps around the urethra as the tube comes out of the bladder. This muscle is always kept tight so pee doesn't leak out when we walk around. The muscle relaxes automatically when a child stands in front of the toilet (boy) or sits (girl or boy) on the toilet. The brain automatically relaxes the external sphincter in this situation. Strong emotion (fear, hearty laughter) can cause the external sphincter to suddenly relax. This initiates a bladder contraction and the bladder totally empties. The child cannot stop the contraction or limit the emptying.

There is no known cure for Giggle Incontinence. There are a variety of common-sense measures to minimize wetting in Giggle

Incontinence. These girls should pee immediately before at-risk social occasions and they should pee frequently during at risk social occasions. These girls should minimize fluid intake during at risk social occasions and then catch up afterwards. These strategies don't prevent the wetting but can minimize the amount of urine. Wearing hoodies and dark-coloured clothes might conceal a wetting episode. Sitting during at risk social occasions is helpful.

Treatment with methylphenidate might help some children with Giggle Incontinence. Since children cannot anticipate the high-risk social situations that trigger an episode, the girl needs to stay on the medication routinely. The family needs to consider whether the episodes are sufficiently frequent and distressing to justify routine use of a medication with potential side effects.

Stress Incontinence

In Stress Incontinence, the bladder only partially empties. The child still has pee left in the bladder when they go to the bathroom immediately after the episode.

Stress Incontinence happens whenever the pressure in the abdomen is increased. The increase in pressure is transmitted to the bladder and sufficient to overcome the muscle tone in the external sphincter and pelvic floor muscles.

Laughter with tickling by a parent, sibling, or friend is often the trigger. Laughter is only one of a variety of common situations that can trigger an episode of Stress Incontinence. Jumping on a trampoline, jumping off a fence, running, contact sports, coughing, sneezing, and playing a trombone or other brass instrument are other causes. Stress Incontinence is more common in preschool and early elementary-aged children and gets less frequent over time as the child learns to anticipate the at-risk situations and tense the pelvic floor muscles to minimize the dampness.

Stool pressure on the bladder increases the risk of Stress Incontinence, so improving bowel health is important. Obesity increases the risk of Stress Incontinence and weight loss reduces the risk.

The conventional treatment is to teach the child Kegel exercises to increase tension in the pelvic floor muscles. I rarely encourage Kegel exercises. Most of the children I see with Stress Incontinence are already keeping their pelvic floor muscles tense to hold in the pee and the poop. I am very reluctant to teach a child to hold in the pee. I only consider this when Stress Incontinence persists later in elementary school, is distressing for the child, and improved bowel health has not resulted in improvement.

Post-void Wetting

Most of the daytime wetting in childhood happens before the child gets to the bathroom. There are four causes of post-void wetting.

Rushing voiding and pulling the pants up
before the bladder has emptied
This is much more common in boys than in girls and more common in busy children with ADHD. Boys should always pull their pants down to make sure the penis is not pulled up and bent over the waist band. Children should allow the stream to completely finish before pulling up the underwear and pants.

Retained pee behind the labia
Girls should mop up any urine that collects behind the labia after a routine void. This prevents the collected urine leaking out when the child pulls up the underwear and pants and walks away. This problem is more common in girls who are overweight.

Retained pee behind the foreskin
Uncircumcised boys might collect some pee behind the foreskin. The drips will leak out when they pull up their underwear and pants to walk away. Mopping up the drips with some tissue will prevent this problem.

Vaginal Reflux of Urine
Some girls with urgency hold their thighs together on the way to the bathroom. With more severe urgency many of these girls "duck waddle" to the bathroom. In this situation the urine comes out and wells up behind the labia which are squeezed tightly together. The

pressure of the urine behind the labia can force the urine into the vagina. This is called vaginal reflux of urine.

In children with vaginal reflux of urine, I see the urine in the vagina when I do an ultrasound before the child voids. When the child pees the urine comes out in two gushes. The first gush is the urine that comes out with the bladder contraction. The second gush is the urine that leaks out of the vaginal as the labia relax apart. Not all of the urine leaks out of the vagina while the child is still sitting on the toilet. A small amount leaks out later when the child pulls up the underwear and clothes, stands up, and walks away.

Bedwetting

Three factors come together to cause bedwetting.

1. The bladder is smaller due to poop pressure.

2. The kidneys make more pee overnight than the smaller bladder can hold.

3. The brain does not wake the child up when the bladder is full.

The first step in the process is the smaller bladder. The other two factors are a consequence of a smaller bladder.

A small bladder changes how a child drinks and this changes how the kidneys make pee over the course of a day

When a bladder is smaller than average this means a child needs to pee more often. Peeing more often is a bother and the child learns to drink less while away from home. Drinking less early in the day changes how the kidneys do their job. The kidneys are a sophisticated filter organ. If a child doesn't drink much early in the day the kidneys do less of their filter function duties early in the day. The solute (chemicals) that needs to be filtered accumulate. If a child doesn't drink much early in the day the hydration suffers and the child gets thirsty later in the day. The child starts to drink when they get home from school. The largest drink of the day is usually the after-school drink. Most of their daily fluid intake happens during a narrow window from home time to after supper. Courtesy of this surge in fluid intake, the accumulated solute is filtered by the kidneys. This results in a surge of pee production overnight. The pee swamps the smaller bladder. Depending on the size of the bladder and the amount of urine produced, the bladder can fill up and empty multiple times. The average number of times a bladder fills up and empties in an early elementary aged child who wets every night is three times. I see children with bladders that fill up and empty as many as 6 times in one night!

Whether a child soaks through the pull up into the bedsheets is an index of how much pee is produced by the kidneys overnight. Soaking through into the bedsheets implies the kidneys make a lot of pee overnight. Poor fit of the pull up and not peeing before bed are other causes. Soaking through into the bedsheets is a real bother and means lots of extra laundry for the mother. Once a child learns to hydrate optimally in the morning before lunch, the daily rhythm of kidney pee production changes. The kidneys make more pee early in the day and process the necessary solute early in the day, and the kidneys make less pee overnight. Once the kidneys make less pee overnight, the laundry problem goes away. Mothers are usually very happy with this change. When a child first attends my clinic I ask the mothers how often the child soaks through the pull up. This can vary from once a month to every night. Every family is instructed to improve morning hydration and not to limit evening fluids. I ask the families to ensure the child drinks water in the evening. When the child returns for the first follow up visit I inquire about the soaking through. If the child is still soaking through with the same frequency, I know the child is not optimally hydrated in the morning. If the soaking through is less or resolved, I point this out to the mother. "So, your child drinks in the evenings but even so, the sheets are dry." Pointing this out helps mothers appreciate the importance of morning hydration.

A small bladder interferes with the ability to wake up to pee

When I ask parents why they think their child wets at night, the most common answer is "He sleeps deep," or "He doesn't wake up." "Yes," I respond, "This is one of the three factors in bedwetting."

When a bladder fills up multiple times every night this implies the bladder fills up from early in the sleep cycle through to the end of the sleep cycle. Sleep is essential for health. Young children especially need their sleep. Sleep interruptions limit quality of sleep. Learning to wake up to pee is difficult enough if you only need to wake up once a night. Learning to wake up to pee twice a night is more difficult. Learning to wake up to pee three times a night is likely not possible. Learning to wake up to pee four or more times is impossible.

As the bladder fills up at night the child experiences a "partial arousal" before the bladder empties. If the parent knew exactly when the child would wet and watched the child in the minutes before the bladder empties, the parent would witness the partial arousal. The child's sleep pattern changes from quiet to restless, the child might talk in their sleep, the child might sit up, or the child might stand up and sleep walk. The child might experience a dream. Night Terrors are sometimes triggered by a full bladder.

About seventy-five percent of children with bedwetting are wet from the start of toilet training. They never achieve night dryness during toilet training. About twenty-five percent of children achieve night dryness during toilet training but later develop bedwetting, most commonly in kindergarten or grade one. In those children who wet right from the start, the size of the bladder was an issue during infancy prior to toilet training. In those who achieved dryness but later started to wet, the bladder became smaller after toilet training. The major factor that causes a small bladder is bowel health. Therefore, bowel health is an issue during infancy in those who are wet from the start. Bowel health during the toddler years is an issue in those who develop bedwetting in the school years.

After toilet training some children only wet the bed intermittently. Children who have dry nights from the start of toilet training have larger bladders than the children who wet every night. When a child has dry nights there are two patterns of dry nights. Either the child sleeps dry with uninterrupted sleep or the child wakes up to pee and sleeps dry. When a child sleeps dry but needs to wake up to pee, this implies the bladder size is a problem because the child should not have to wake up to pee. The ability to wake to pee implies the bladder size is likely fifty to seventy-five percent of average and the bladder fills up once later in the sleep cycle when waking up to pee is easier. On dry nights when a child sleeps dry and does not need to wake to pee, the amount of pee made overnight by the kidneys fits in the bladder. On these nights the bladder size is likely at least seventy-five percent of average. On wet nights the bladder size is likely less than fifty percent of average and the bladder fills up multiple times, including early in the sleep cycle when waking to pee is more difficult. I point these patterns out to the parents to help them appreciate the relationship of bladder size to the ability to wake up to pee.

In children who are dry at night immediately after toilet training and who develop bedwetting later, usually around kindergarten or grade one, the bladder size was adequate after toilet training and got smaller over time. When a child was dry but needed to wake up to pee to sleep dry, the ability to wake up to pee is eventually lost as the bladder starts to fill up earlier and earlier in the sleep cycle and more than one time each night. When a child with secondary onset bedwetting woke up to pee as a toddler, I point this out to the parents. I reassure the parents that since their child could wake up to pee, the skill will return once the bladder is bigger.

Interventions that don't work to cure bedwetting

Limiting fluids after supper

Most parents limit fluids in the evening. Not only does this not work, but this is part of the reason why bowel health is such a problem. One of the basic principles I teach is that hydration is important for health and the goal is a child who is dry and able to hydrate in the evenings for sports and social activities.

Taking the child to pee when the parents go to bed

This intervention can result in dry nights in a child who has a bladder size that is at least fifty to seventy-five percent of average but does not cure the problem. Still, dry nights are an ego boost and sometimes this intervention allows a child to sleep dry and not wear a pull up, which is another ego boost. However, this intervention does not cure the problem. Many parents presume taking their child to pee when the parent goes to bed or setting an alarm and taking their child to pee at set times overnight will teach their child to wake to pee on their own. This doesn't happen. The reason why this doesn't happen is because a child needs to learn to wake up to pee WHEN THE BLADDER IS FULL. The brain needs to learn to wake the child at a precise moment, the moment when the pressure receptors in the bladder send a signal to the brain that the bladder is full. When a parent randomly takes a child to pee, the bladder is not full, and there is no opportunity for the brain to learn.

Stopping the pull-up

Many parents experiment with stopping the pull up. The hope is that the child will start to wake up to pee rather than suffer sleeping in wet sheets. If the bladder is at least fifty to seventy-five percent of average and therefore fills only once overnight later in the sleep cycle, this intervention has a chance of success. If a parent would like to try this intervention I recommend the family improve bowel health first so the bladder is bigger. Once the bowel health and bladder size are clearly improved I recommend the family discuss this intervention with the child and set a date to stop wearing the pull up. The family should talk this up in the days or weeks before the event so the child is thinking about waking to pee. The child needs to understand that waking to pee is about waking up and not about feeling like you need to pee. Many children wake up with a full bladder but don't feel like they need to pee. The feeling is different lying down and coming out of sleep. The parents should set up a reward for waking to pee (not for dryness).

Rewards

Parents often offer rewards in the hope that a child will be dry to obtain the reward. This approach presumes a child has control and can "decide" to be dry. This is not the case. Bedwetting is due to a small bladder, too much pee, and not waking up. The child has no control over these factors and rewards for dryness per se will not usually help.

Treatment of Bedwetting

Bedwetting is caused by three factors.

1. The bladder is smaller due to poop pressure

2. The kidneys make more pee overnight than the smaller bladder can hold.

3. The brain does not wake the child up when the bladder is full.

To achieve dryness at night you need to work on all three factors. You need to work on the three factors in the correct sequence. Until the bladder size improves and the overnight kidney pee production decreases such that the bladder only fills up and empties once or maximum twice a night, there is no sense working on learning to wake to pee. Learning to wake to pee is therefore the last factor to work on.

Working on the three factors requires changes in behaviour. Changing behaviour takes time and practice. Most families will need a minimum of six months to achieve dryness. To improve bladder size and reduce overnight pee production takes about three months. Learning to wake up to pee takes another three months.

I tell all the families that my behavioural approach works but that my approach is WORK. Life conspires against about a third of the families who attend my clinic and they are not able to follow the recommendations and achieve success. Many return a few years later when their lives are less complicated and try again with success.

Increasing the size of the bladder is all about improving bowel health and letting some time pass. Time is a factor. With improved bowel health the bladder needs time and practice to "learn" to hold more.

The bladder in a newborn only holds about 50 ml. With the rapid growth in infancy, the bladder can hold 175 ml by two years. Thereafter the bladder slowly increases in size by about 25 ml per year. A six-year-old bladder should hold 275 ml. A ten-year-old bladder should hold 350 ml.

When a child wets every night, this implies the bladder is less than fifty percent of the average size for age. Children with one or more dry nights each week usually have a bladder size that is fifty to seventy-five percent of average for age. Night dryness slowly improves with age because the bladder slowly gets bigger with age. The bladder gets bigger because the pelvis slowly gets bigger and there is more room for the bladder and the effect of bowel health is relatively less. Bedwetting often finally resolves after the pubertal growth spurt, presumably because the pelvic volume increases and there is relatively more room for the bladder.

The magic number for the size of a bladder such that a child can learn to wake up to pee is about 200 ml. When the bladder is about this size the bladder will only fill up once or twice a night and learning to wake up to pee is a practical possibility.

At the first visit to my clinic, I explain the bedwetting factors and I review the three bowel health goals to achieve Bladder Friendly Bowel Health. Once the child achieves these goals I reassess the child. I confirm the goals have been achieved. Then I measure the bladder size by collecting two weeks of overnight pee measurements. If the first morning voided volume data confirms the bladder can hold at least 200 ml of pee, then I discuss learning to wake up to pee. Learning to wake up to pee requires a bedwetting alarm for a minimum of three months.

Alarm Therapy

Four goals of bedwetting alarm therapy

1. Child is dry and no longer wearing a pull up

2. Child learns to wake up to pee

3. Size of the bladder increases into the average range for age.

4. Child can overhydrate in the evening and still be dry.

The success rate to achieve these four goals in my clinic is eighty to ninety percent. I help families through the alarm process with regular visits to my clinic. At each visit I outline a new set of goals and exercises to practice until the next visit. A typical schedule is a coaching session the day the child starts alarm therapy. The first follow up is in two weeks. Thereafter there are monthly follow ups until the child achieves all four goals. The decision to stop is based on achievement of all four goals. Seventy-five percent of families need three months; about twenty-five percent require an extra month. Occasionally alarm therapy takes more than four months.

Setting up the alarm

I recommend an alarm with a sensor that can be attached to cotton underwear the child wears under the pull up. A sensor attached to the underwear will result in an alarm with the first drops of pee. I do not recommend a mattress alarm since the alarm will not be triggered by the first drops of pee. The cotton underwear should be snug briefs and not floppy boxer style.

At the coaching session I explain how the alarm works. I demonstrate how one drop of water (urine) can trigger the alarm.

I ask the child to wear the alarm clipped to the shoulder on a t-shirt, pajamas, or nightie. The alarm needs to be close to the ear so the noise is loud and annoying.

The sensor clip should be placed in the midline on the cotton underwear by the parent. The clip should be positioned as close as possible to where the urine is expected to come out. The parent should examine the underwear after each alarm and adjust the clip position as necessary to achieve the most precise placement.

The electrical cord from the alarm to the sensor should be under the t-shirt pajama top or nightie. This prevents the arm of a child getting tangled in the cord.

Hearing the alarm

The parent must be able to hear the alarm. The parent and the child should be on the same floor. With the bedroom doors both open, about seventy-five percent of parents can hear the alarm. If the parent cannot hear the alarm, then either a baby monitor should be put in the room of the child, or the parent and the child should sleep in the same room.

Sleeping in the same room has advantages apart from hearing the alarm. Sleeping in the same room is a solidarity gesture. This confirms the parent is invested in the process. For younger, less mature children, and for children with anxiety, the presence of the parent can make a big difference. If the parent does choose to sleep in the same room, this should only be temporary. The child and the parent need to relocate back to their respective bedrooms. I usually try to achieve this by two weeks and at the latest by six weeks.

Many parents are concerned the alarm will wake up other family members. This might be a problem in the first week but thereafter the rest of the family sleeps through, even surprisingly when a sibling shares the same bedroom.

Some parents have problems waking up because of medications, sleep apnea, or other sleep disorders. In this situation another caregiver needs to be recruited (the other parent, grandparent, older adolescent sibling).

Turning off the Alarm

Only a parent should turn off the alarm. The child should be specifically instructed not to turn off the alarm.

The Three Steps to Learn to Wake up to Pee

1. Alertness
2. Stopping the pee
3. Beating the buzzer

First Step is Alertness

Alertness is the first step. This is the responsibility of the parent. The parent must wake the child to the alert, fully awake state of consciousness.

After the parent hears the alarm, the parent needs to arrive **promptly** at the bedside of the child. The parent needs to help the child wake up. **The parent should not turn off the alarm until the parent is convinced the child is fully awake.** This might take a few minutes. The parent should get the child sitting with their legs over the side of the bed. The parent should make sure the child has good eye contact and can answer questions coherently. Once this is achieved the parent should turn off the alarm. Every morning the parent needs to question the child to determine if the child can recollect the alarm, getting up, and something the child and parent talked about. If the child cannot remember, the child was not fully alert and the next night the parent should spend more time and effort to wake the child to the fully alert state of consciousness. Sometimes this requires walking the child around the room. Cool clothes on the face or drinking a few ounces of cold water might help. The most common alertness pattern is for the child to take three or four nights to become fully alert and to consistently remember the next morning. Once this is achieved the parent should continue to spend the necessary time to wake the child and should always check the next morning. A parent should not presume that a child who can carry on a conversation or a child who can walk on their own to the bathroom is fully alert. Sometimes the child is sleep talking and sleep walking. Remembering the next morning is very important.

Alertness is a bigger concern when alarms go off early in the sleep cycle. A parent might need to spend more time waking the child when alarms occur before or around midnight.

Second Step is Stop the Pee

The second step is for the child to stop the pee. This is the child's main responsibility. As soon as the child hears the alarm, the child needs to tense the pelvic floor muscles and stop the pee. The goal is to stop the pee so fast that the pee does not get into the pull up. The child needs to limit the pee to the underwear.

I ask the child to demonstrate they know how to stop the pee while in the office. While with the parent in the bathroom, I ask the parent to instruct the child to "stop" the pee for second and then instruct the child to "start" the pee. I ask the parent to do this several times. Most children know how to stop the pee. If they seem confused, I ask them to "squeeze their bum cheeks" to stop the pee. The child needs to practice stopping the pee at home. I ask the child to practice with every void. While they practice, I ask the child to "talk to your brain, tell your brain what you want to do." Practice makes perfect. I ask the child to strive to stop the pee ninety percent of alarms. Stopping the pee is a very important skill.

I ask the parent to score the ability of their child to stop the pee. When the child is excellent at stopping the pee and the pee is limited to the underwear, this is scored a "1." When some pee goes through into the pull-up, this is scored a "2." When the pull-up is filled with a lot of pee, much like a routine wetting, this is a "3." I ask the child to practice until they are "number 1." When a child stops the pee with a "1," the amount of pee voided into the toilet after the alarm is a good estimate of the average bladder volume. With a "2" there is pee in the pull-up and less pee voided into the toilet. With a "3" there is a lot of pee in the pull-up and little or no urine to void into the toilet. Children usually start with a "3," improve to a "2," and then start to achieve "1."

Third Step is Beat the Buzzer

After the child is consistently alert and is consistent at stopping the pee, the brain automatically starts to wake the child before the bladder empties, before the child wets the bed, before the alarm goes off. I call this Beating the Buzzer.

The learning (conditioning) scenario I envision is that the brain recognizes that the child does not like the loud annoying noise. The brain recognizes that the child is trying to stop the pee coming out. The brain recognizes that the child does not want to wet the bed. Based on this information, the brain does the right thing to solve the problem and wakes the child up. Waking the child up prevents the annoying noise. Waking the child up ensures the pee stops. Waking the child up helps the child achieve the desired goal of dryness.

I instruct the child that Beating the Buzzer is about waking up and not about feeling like you need to pee. This is an important point. The bladder does not routinely feel full when a child Beats the Buzzer. Without this instruction, a tired child might roll over and fall back asleep. Ouch. Missed opportunity. Going in the wrong direction.

When a child Beats the Buzzer, they need to get out of bed, go to the parent, and wake the parent. The parent should congratulate the child and make this a big deal. Then the child should pee. Then the parent puts the alarm back on and tucks the child back into bed.

Some families who come to my clinic tried a bedwetting alarm and were not successful. When I inquire about their past experience the parents report two common reasons for failure.

1. The child didn't wake. This is why I teach the parent to arrive promptly at the bedside and for the parent to wake the child to full alert consciousness. Waking the child is the job of the parent.

2. The child turned off the alarm and went back to sleep. This is why I teach only the parent should turn off the alarm. If the child does turn off the alarm the parent needs to sleep in the same room to prevent this.

Goals for the First Two Weeks

1. The child achieves consistent alertness.
2. The child is able to stop the pee and the trend to consistency is improving.

Scenarios for first two weeks

Typical Scenario

The typical or average scenario is present in about sixty-five to seventy-five percent of children on alarm therapy. The typical scenario predicts success with continued efforts.

A parent will take 3 or 4 days working on alertness before the child remembers. Thereafter the child will mostly remember except for alarms early in the sleep cycle. Thereafter the parent will still need to be vigilant but alertness is usually fine.

The child will stop the pee and limit the pee to the underwear during the first week, usually around the time the alertness is good and after a few days of daytime practice. The ability to stop the pee is more consistent in the second week because the child is more alert and because the child continues to practice and think about this important skill during the day. The parent needs to remind the child to practice during the day.

There are no beat the buzzers in the first two weeks. The alertness and stopping the pee skills are not yet consistent enough.

When the parent arrives at the bedside, the child is lying down and not getting up. The child is "waiting" on the parent for help to get up. The child is tired. If the parent does not arrive promptly at the bedside, the child might fall back asleep while the alarm is going, which is not good.

There are usually two alarms a night in the first week and one alarm a night in the second week. Both the parent and child are tired. The parent is more tired because the parent often doesn't fall back asleep as quickly, but the tiredness is manageable.

Best Case Scenario

The best-case scenario happens in twenty to twenty-five percent of children. This scenario predicts success.

In this scenario the child is alert from the first night. The parent is able to turn the alarm off within a minute and the child remembers well the next morning.

The child stops the pee the first or second night and there is a trend to more consistency by the end of the first week and this improves again in the second week.

There is a beat the buzzer in the first two weeks!

When the parent arrives at the bedside the child is getting up on their own. They are lifting their head off the bed. By the end of the first week the child is sitting up. By the end of the second week the child is standing up and perhaps meeting the parent in the doorway or hall.

There are two alarms a night in the first week and one in the second. Tiredness is manageable.

Worst Case Scenario

The worst-case scenario happens in only five percent of children. This scenario does not predict success.

In this scenario the parent reports the child is very difficult to wake up. The parent spends increasing time to wake the child but remembering is intermittent or not present. Parents spend up to a maximum of fifteen minutes walking the child around, use cold clothes on the face, ask the child to drink a few ounces of cold water, all to no avail. The child does not stop the pee or beat the buzzer. When the parent arrives at the bedside the child is sleeping soundly and there is no response to the alarm. This scenario does not predict success and I usually recommend stopping alarm therapy.

Goals for Two to Six weeks

1. The child continues to practice alertness and stopping the pee.
2. The child stops wearing the pull up.
3. The child beats the buzzer.
4. The average bladder volume increases.
5. The child might be able to start the overhydration practice and drink more water in the evening.

Stopping the Pee Practice

Skill at stopping the pee is important early in alarm therapy because this is part of the alertness conditioning that leads to beating the buzzer.

Skill at stopping the pee is also important at the end of alarm therapy. The relapse rate is lower in children who have excellent stop the pee skills.

If stopping the pee is not consistent the parent needs to remind the child to practice stopping the pee with every void during the day and especially with the before bed void. The child needs to practice and think about stopping the pee while awake during the day.

If the child has problems stopping the pee, I prescribe specific exercises to practice three times a day. The parent and child work together to practice tensing the pelvic floor muscles while awake and when the bladder is not full. The parent instructs the child to tense the pelvic floor muscles and hold the tension for a count of five. The parent instructs the child to do five sets of these exercises three times a day. The parent needs to supervise the exercises.

Stopping the Pull up

Excellence at stopping the pee is how a child EARNS the right to stop wearing a pull up. The child needs to stop the pee a minimum of four alarms in a row. Note, this is four alarms and not four nights in a row. Some children sleep dry or beat the buzzer in between alarms. Once the child stops the pee four alarms in a row, the child needs to consider the decision to stop wearing the pull up. The responsibility to stop wearing the pull up **needs to be made by the child**. The child needs to feel confident and ready to take this step. The rule is that once you stop wearing the pull up you NEVER go back. Most children are keen to stop wearing the pull up but a few are reluctant to make this step.

Beating the Buzzer

The child usually starts to beat the buzzer between two to six weeks on alarm therapy. This usually happens after several weeks of consistent alertness and when the child achieves stopping the pee skills that are consistent and around ninety percent of alarms. Sometimes beating the buzzer starts within the first few nights after the child stops wearing the pull up.

Once the child starts to beat the buzzer the parent celebrates and talks about this achievement. To motivate the child, the parent should consider a reward for every subsequent beat the buzzer.

Average Bladder Volume Increases

If the poop is soft and the first morning poop routine is established, the average bladder volume slowly increases on alarm therapy. The average bladder volume is the volume when the child beats the buzzer or stops the pee and limits the pee to the underwear (STP score = 1). The average bladder volume usually increases by about 25 to 50 ml a month.

As the average bladder volume increases the number of alarms decrease. As the average bladder volume increases the time when either the alarm occurs or when the child wakes and beats the buzzer happens later and later in the sleep cycle. As the average bladder volume increases the child might begin to sleep dry without the occurrence of either an alarm or a beat the buzzer. I call this **Sleeping Dry**. Sleeping dry is NOT a beat the buzzer. The first AM voided volume in a child who sleeps dry should not be used to assess average bladder volume. The sleeping dry volume is usually higher than the average bladder volume. The bladder can hold more when the bladder fills slowly over the entire night.

Overhydration Practice

One of the four goals of alarm therapy is the ability to drink extra water and still be dry. Extra water is more water than the child would otherwise drink based on thirst, activity, or socialization. Drinking extra water is a "test" of dryness. Overhydration practice helps a child to be more confident in their ability to sleep dry.

Once there is only one wake up (alarm or beat the buzzer) a night, and once the child is no longer wearing a pull up, the child needs to start to drink extra water in the evening before bed. The parent should set a smart phone alarm for one hour before bed. When the alarm goes off, the parent should get some water for the child to drink. The child is obliged to drink even if they are not thirsty. The mother should start with 125 ml and go up slowly and methodically by 25 ml a week.

Goals for Six to Ten Weeks

1. Continued practice with alertness and stopping the pee.
2. Continued practice beating the buzzer.
3. Average bladder volume increases.
4. Overhydration practice.

The last half of alarm therapy is about practice. The skill set of alertness, stopping the pee, and beating the buzzer should be established. The child should not be wearing the pull up. If the child is reluctant to stop wearing the pull up I encourage the child to make this step. They need to make this decision before they stop alarm therapy. The bladder volume should slowly increase. The child should slowly increase how much they drink in the evening.

Beating the Buzzer Practice

The goal is for the child to beat the buzzer at least 25 times before the end of alarm therapy. This is one reason why alarm therapy sometimes needs an extra fourth month. The child needs practice with this essential skill.

There are almost always alarms right until the end of alarm therapy. Ideally there should be only about one alarm a week at the end of alarm therapy. I am not concerned about one alarm a week so long as the child can stop the pee and can beat the buzzer. Very few children are "perfect" and have no alarms and only beat the buzzer by the end of alarm therapy. It is helpful for the child and parents to know this.

Some children become complacent and allow the alarm to get them up. The parent needs to encourage the child to **turn the alarms into beat the buzzers**. Ideally each week there should a slow improvement in the ratio of alarms to beat the buzzers. I challenge the parent and child to "work" the ratio of alarms to beat the buzzers. I ask the parent to motivate the child with encouragement and rewards. The child should be offered a negotiated reward for each beat the buzzer. Each week the parent and child should look at the pattern and establish a new goal and revise the incentive. Make this a game. The child should continue to be rewarded for every beat the buzzer. If the child improves the number of beat the buzzers during the week the child should receive an extra reward. I call this "working the ratio of alarms to beat the buzzers."

Average Bladder Volume Increase

At every visit I ask the child to sit after breakfast to poop, to sustain great morning hydration and to stay on the stool softener. The average bladder volume will only increase if the poop is soft. If the average bladder volume does not improve this is a reason to continue on alarm therapy for an extra month.

Overhydration Practice

The amount of water the child drinks one hour before bed should slowly increase. Most children will eventually drink 250 to 360 ml of extra water.

The slow increase in the extra water insures the child will not sleep dry and will get the necessary practice beating the buzzer. The slow increase in the extra water helps the bladder to learn to hold more.

Goals for Ten to Twelve Weeks

Once all four goals are achieved, then the child stops drinking the extra water and "coasts" to the end of alarm therapy. Since there is less water in the evenings, the number of alarms or beat the buzzers is less and the child sleeps dry more often. After these two weeks of "coasting," now three months on the alarm, the child stops wearing the alarm.

Monitoring during alarm therapy

When I help families through alarm therapy, I ask them to track some basic data to help me guide them better.

Figure 1 shows the data I recommend the family collect each day the child is on alarm therapy. Starting from the first column on the left is the day of the week and then the day of the month. The next two columns are to record the time of the daily poops. I never stop talking about the goal to achieve and sustain a soft first morning poop and a second poop later in the day. The next two columns are to record Beat the Buzzer data. The parent should record the time and the volume of urine voided by the child with the Beat the Buzzer. The next four columns are for the first alarm of the night. The parent should record the time, whether a child remembers getting up with the alarm (parent asks and records this the next morning), how well the child stopped the pee (score 1 or 2 or 3), and the volume of urine voided when the child gets up with the alarm. The next four columns are for the second alarm of the night. The next column is the volume of urine when the child wakes up in the morning. The child must pee even if they don't feel like they need to pee. The final column is the Total Volume, which is the sum of all the wake-up pees, which includes the amount left after an alarm, the Beat the Buzzer volume, and the first morning volume. The data in the calendar tells the story of the child's progress.

Figure 2 shows the data I recommend once the child has made progress and there is only one alarm a night. Typically, this will be at the two or six week follow-up. Figure 2 only has room to enter one alarm a night. Figure 2 has a column at the far right to record how much a child drinks after supper. This column records progress with overhydration practice.

The average bladder volume is estimated by calculating the average of the volumes when a child wakes with a beat the buzzer. Another estimate of the average bladder volume is the average of the volumes when a child stops the pee and limits the pee to the underwear. Both these situations allow a good estimate of the average bladder volume during the time since the last clinic visit. Typically, the average bladder volume slowly improves over alarm therapy. The sleep dry first morning voided volume is not a good estimate of the average volume.

Once a child is consistent at stopping the pee, the Total Volume represents the amount of pee produced overnight by the kidneys. This is an important number to track. If the Total Volume is too high, there will be too many alarms and the child and parent might tire out, and alarm therapy might not be successful. If the Total Volume is too low, there are too few alarms, and the child will not get sufficient practice stopping the pee or beating the buzzer, and the bladder will not learn to hold more. After the child starts the overhydration practice, the Total Volume goes up as the amount the child drinks in the evening goes up.

Figure 1

Day	Date	1st Poop Time	2nd Poop Time	BTB Time	Volume	Alarm Time	Memory Y N	STP 3 2 1	Volume	Alarm Time	Memory Y N	STP 3 2 1	Volume	First AM Volume	Total Volume
Mon															
Tue															
Wed															
Thu															
Fri															
Sat															
Sun															

Figure 2

Day	Date	1st Poop Time	2nd Poop Time	Alarm Time	Memory Y N	STP 3 2 1	Volume	BTB Time	Volume	First AM Volume	Total Volume	Drink Eve oz
Mon												
Tue												
Wed												
Thu												
Fri												
Sat												
Sun												

Troubleshooting Common Problems on Alarm Therapy

Alarm therapy when there are two homes and shared custody

Consistency is necessary for success. Unless there is excellent communication and cooperation between the two homes I don't recommend alarm therapy.

Travelling during alarm therapy

I do not recommend travel during alarm therapy, especially during the first half (six weeks) when the skill set is established. Travelling interferes with consistency. Travel in the last half, once the skill set is established, is less problematic. Travel mostly prolongs alarm therapy.

Sports evenings on alarm therapy

Evening sports increases the challenges on alarm therapy. A tired child might not wake as easily. Children under or overhydrate on sports nights. Notwithstanding these factors, I prefer a child to play their customary evening sport on alarm therapy. Playing sports is important for child development. A child needs to learn to be dry and play their chosen sport. Hydration on a sports night sometimes requires management. The Total Volume is a good guide to whether child needs to increase or decrease the hydration with the sport.

Fever and respiratory infection while on alarm therapy

If a child develops a fever and respiratory symptoms, or any significant illness that keeps them home from school, I recommend the parent pause alarm therapy and allow the child to rest until they resume school attendance.

Too many alarms

When there are too many alarms each night either the child or the parent will wear out and progress will stall or the project will fail.

Most families can tolerate up to two alarms for a few weeks and one alarm or beat the buzzer wake up thereafter. Three or more alarms in the first two weeks or more than two alarms thereafter is too much for most parents and children to manage.

Too many alarms usually happens because the bowel health is not optimal. The child is still missing days. The child did not establish a first AM poop pattern. The poop is still pasty or hard.

Temporary interventions while the family works to improve bowel health include taking the child to pee when the parent goes to bed (reduces one wake up for the parent) and reducing fluids with supper or in the evening after supper. I only use these interventions to buy some time and only if I sense the situation will be temporary. These interventions are "steps back" and always prolong the time on alarm therapy beyond three months.

In some children the bowel health is satisfactory and the bladder size is still a concern. If I am convinced the bowel health is bladder-friendly I consider prescribing oxybutynin. This medication can increase bladder size but only if the bladder is surrounded by soft poop. I prescribe this medication for a month or two and always stop the medication before the child stops alarm therapy.

Child does not learn to beat the buzzer

Alertness and stopping the pee are pre-requisites for learning to beat the buzzer. Parents need to be consistent and disciplined waking a child to full alert consciousness. The child need to practice stopping the pee with each void during the day and the child needs to think about how much they want to stop the pee when the alarm goes off. Some children only start to beat the buzzer after they stop wearing the pull up.

Some children are alert, can stop the pee, and have stopped wearing a pull up and still do not beat the buzzer. I teach these children a "visualization" exercise, a "get out of bed to pee" exercise. Once a day, when at home, and when the child has a full bladder they need to practice this exercise. When the bladder is full they ask a parent to help. They go into their room and lie down on the bed in their typical sleep position (side, back, tummy, hugging a pillow or stuffy). Then they close their eyes. Then the parent turns out the light. Now the child is in bed, in their typical sleep position, with eyes closed, and the bladder is full. This is exactly the situation just before the alarm goes off at night. I ask the child to think about how much they want to be dry, about how much they want to beat the buzzer. After thinking about this in bed the child gets up and walks to the bathroom. As the child walks to the bathroom, the child "talks" to his brain and tells the brain this is what I want to do tonight.

Motivation helps. The parents need to talk about beating the buzzer. The parents should offer a reward for every time the child beats the buzzer. One family offered their boy a "signed" Calgary Flame's jersey if he beat the buzzer! He beat the buzzer two nights in a row, got his jersey, then promptly resumed wetting. Ouch. Parents should change up the rewards sufficiently to sustain motivation. The best reward should be the satisfaction of a job well done.

Progress stalls

A stall pattern is present when a child continues to experience alarms and does not make progress converting alarms to beat the buzzers. More than two alarms a week during the last month on alarm therapy is a variation of stalled progress.

There are three causes of the stall pattern.

1. Tiredness

2. Discouragement

3. Complacency

Tiredness happens when there are too many alarms, when the child is not getting enough sleep otherwise, when sports events wear out the child, and when there are intercurrent stresses at home or school that affect sleep quality. Improving sleep duration and quality help.

Discouragement happens when the initial keenness to work on dryness wears off and the child realizes alarm therapy is a lot of work and dryness is not immediate. Motivation suffers.

Complacency happens when a child does very well and acquires the skill set for success but thereafter lets the alarms get them up rather than working to convert alarms to beat the buzzers.

If I can motivate a discouraged or complacent child, the progress will resume. If I cannot motivate the child, alarm therapy might not be successful.

How to Sustain Dryness

Once a child achieves the four alarm therapy goals and stops the alarm, I spend one more session to discuss how to sustain dryness. I review the progress since the first visit and find ways to congratulate the child on their achievement. Then I tell the child they are dry because they achieved three things and they need to continue to work on these three things.

1. The child learned how to wake up to pee.

2. They learned that bladder size is related to great bowel health.

3. They learned that morning hydration is important to ensure the kidneys make pee in an optimal daily rhythm.

The child needs to continue to practice waking to pee. If they do not wake to pee at least once a week on their own, the parent needs to trigger the need to wake to pee with extra evening fluids once a week. I recommend once a week practice for the next year. I tell the child to be disciplined. They can lose the wake the pee skill if they do not routinely get out of bed to pee whenever they wake up. I tell them to "Use it or lose it." I tell them never to wear a pull up again.

The child needs to sustain the bladder-friendly bowel health pattern. I tell them to stay on the softener for three more months and after they stop the softener to monitor the bowel health and use the softener intermittently as necessary if the poop pattern gets worse.

The child needs to always carry their water bottle at school and continue to drink lots before lunch.

Reasons for Failure

Only about ten percent of children in my clinic do not achieve dryness. The most common reason is the bladder is too small, mostly because the bowel health was not bladder-friendly. The second most common reason Is the child did not cooperate with alarm therapy. The third most common reason is the child did not learn to stop the pee or beat the buzzer. The fourth most common reason is the parent did not follow the rules or otherwise gave up.

Relapses

Relapses happen in about ten percent of children who achieve dryness. Most relapses occur within the first year. A relapse is defined as bedwetting with a soaker and the child does not wake up with the episode. If this happens once a week for several weeks, this is sufficient to consider a relapse. Relapses usually respond to another course of alarm therapy. Most relapses occur because the bowel health gets worse again, the bladder gets smaller, and the bladder starts to fill up earlier in the sleep cycle when waking to pee is more difficult.

Dysfunctional Voiding

Dysfunctional Voiding is a specific diagnostic category recognized by the International Children's Continence Society (ICCS). To qualify for this diagnosis a child needs to have poor bladder emptying, difficulty relaxing the external sphincter, and no evidence of a neurogenic bladder. The bladder wall is usually thick and irregular. There is usually a history of urinary tract infection. Constipation and soiling are common. The condition is chronic.

Early reports of this condition used the moniker non-neurogenic neurogenic bladder because poor bladder emptying and failure to relax the external sphincter is common in neurogenic bladder, but in Dysfunctional Voiding there is no evidence of a nerve abnormality of the lumbar spine. Dr. Frank Hinman, one of the fathers of Paediatric Urology in the United States reported on this problem and some still refer to the condition as Hinman's Syndrome. I prefer the generic description, Dysfunctional Voiding. I don't use the term very often. Rather, in keeping with my philosophy to think about and discuss symptoms and signs rather than to use diagnostic labels, I think about this condition as a problem with bladder emptying and a problem with relaxation of the external sphincter.

Failure to Empty the Bladder

The bladder is a simple organ with two basic functions. The bladder needs to fill up and the bladder needs to empty.

In health, the bladder can empty to leave only drips of urine, less than one ml. The bladder is designed to empty without the need for any external push by the child.

The most common cause of poor emptying is an overfull bladder. As soon as a child holds the pee past full, the bladder muscles are "stressed" and emptying is compromised. The term that describes the volume of urine that remains after voiding is post-void-residual. If the child goes a little past full, the post-void-residual might be up to 5 ml (one teaspoon). If the child goes past full sufficiently to develop urgency, the post-void-residual will be higher, perhaps 5 to 10 ml. If the child has severe urgency or squatting, the post-void-residual will be higher, perhaps up to 15 to 30 ml.

I do a uroflow study whenever a child voids in my clinic. The child is instructed to pee into a special toilet that has a pressure sensitive device that measures the volume of pee voided. The uroflow curve also demonstrates the force of the bladder contraction during the void. A normal uroflow curve with a bladder that is just full (relaxed) is a symmetrical bell shape. A uroflow curve in a child who holds the pee past full is lower and wider with a tower-shape. A uroflow curve in a child with urgency and dampness is even lower and wider. A wide low uroflow curve is an obstructive curve. The curves get lower and wider because a child with an overfull bladder keeps the pelvic floor muscles tense to hold in the pee and this creates a relative obstruction to the flow of urine.

The table below shows the correlations between bladder fullness, bladder muscle tension, post-void residual volume, and the uroflow shape. The table applies to acute changes in fullness as might happen void by void in a child who holds the urine past full intermittently over the course of a day.

Bladder Fullness	Bladder Muscle	Post-void Residual	Uroflow Curve Shape
Full	Relaxed	0 to 1 ml	Bell
A bit overfull	Past Relaxed	2 to 5 ml	Bell-Tower
Overfull with urgency	Stressed	6 to 15 ml	Tower
Overfull with severe urgency, dampness.	Very Stressed	16 to 30 ml or more	Broad

In a child who habitually holds the pee past full, bladder emptying might be permanently compromised. In this situation, the ability to empty is lost even at modest bladder volumes and pressures. This takes years of chronic overfilling and high pressure. Dysfunctional voiding is likely the end result of chronically high bladder pressures.

The bladder wall thickness in these children is wider than normal. The bladder wall in a child who does not hold the pee past full is less than three mm. I regularly measure bladder wall thickness up to five mm in children who hold the pee past full and I have measured bladder wall thickness as high as nine mm.

Once the bladder chronically loses the ability to empty, bladder infections start to play a role in the voiding problems, even in boys.

Failure to Relax the External Sphincter

The bladder muscle and the external sphincter muscle are controlled by different nerves from the spinal cord. The external sphincter muscle is designed to stay tense until the moment when a child decides to pee. Once the child is in the bathroom and ready to pee, the brain sends a signal to the external sphincter to relax. Urine starts to come out of the bladder and the bladder muscles automatically contract to empty the bladder.

Failure to relax the external sphincter muscle plays a role in the failure to empty in a child with Dysfunctional Voiding. If the external sphincter does not relax, this creates a relative obstruction to the flow of urine. The uroflow curve is lower and wider and the bladder does not empty totally. When the external sphincter relaxes erratically, the uroflow curve is interrupted. In children with Dysfunctional Voiding, the tension in the external sphincter stays erratically high during voiding.

Treatment of Dysfunctional Voiding

The first step is to achieve bladder-friendly bowel health and take the pressure of the poop pushing into the bladder.

I believe that the poor emptying and failure to relax the external sphincter can be improved with bladder physiotherapy.

The underlying treatment principle is to keep the bladder pressure low. The child needs to learn to pee more often at smaller volumes. The child needs to learn to get in touch with the early signals of fullness and to respond promptly.

I perform a sufficient number of uroflow and post void residual measurements in my clinic to identify the optimal bladder volume for the child to void. The optimal volume has the best emptying and most normal uroflow curve. Invariably at the first assessment the child routinely voids with much higher (overfull) volumes on a routine basis. I ask the child to pee "sooner" or I ask the child to void randomly after a drinking a lot. After I collect sufficient data, I prepare a table to review with the parent.

Child's Perception of Fullness	Voided Volume	Post-void-Residual	Uroflow Curve Shape
Not Full	100 ml	4 ml	Bell
Not Full	150 ml	6 ml	Bell
Not Full	200 ml	11 ml	Bell-Tower
"Kinda" Full	225 ml	15 ml	Tower
Overfull with urgency	250 ml	30 ml	Tower-Broad
Overfull with severe urgency, damp	275 ml	60 ml	Broad

In the scenario in the table, this child empties the bladder best at volumes of 100 to 150 ml. After this volume the post-void residual is too high and the uroflow curve deteriorates (lower and wider). I review this with the parent and recommend that the parent work at least once a week at home for an afternoon or morning to practice peeing at smaller volumes in the range of 100 to 150 ml. The parent asks the child to drink enough water to need to pee. The child is instructed to pee as soon as they feel the signal. The parent measures the volume voided. If the volumes are more than 150 ml the parent repeats the drink-and-pee-sooner instruction and again measures the voided volume. With practice the child can learn to pee at smaller volumes. Over months this will improve the symptoms of urgency and daytime dampness. With further time and practice the abnormal uroflow curve and emptying start to improve. This takes months and sometimes years.

Bladder Infection

Bladder infection (cystitis) causes the bladder to feel full at a smaller volume and this results in voiding frequently. Bladder infection also compromises bladder control and this results in urgency and daytime wetting.

Bladder infection is predominantly a problem in girls. The traditional reason offered to explain why girls are more susceptible is that the female urethra is shorter than the male urethra.

The bacteria that cause bladder infection usually live in the gastrointestinal tract where they perform a variety of useful functions. However, in the urinary tract they cause infection. The traditional explanation to explain the presence of gastrointestinal bacteria in the urinary tract is that the gastrointestinal bacteria hang out in the genital area and "climb" up the urethra into the bladder.

Situations that Increase the Risk of Bladder Infection

1. Any situation that increases the number of gastrointestinal bacteria in the genital region

2. Situations that increase the risk of uncommon bacteria in the genital region.

Situations that increase the number of gastrointestinal bacteria in the genital region

A common risk factor is wiping the wrong way (back to front) after a poop. The child should be taught to wipe front to back so the bacteria are wiped away from the urethra.

Another common risk factor is not promptly changing a soiled diaper or clothes.

A diaper or genital rash is a risk factor.

Labial fusion is a risk factor. This is a problem in infant girls. There is sufficient inflammation in the genital region that the labia fuse together. This creates a pocket where "stagnant" urine can collect.

Situations that increase the exposure to uncommon bacteria in the genital tract

Our body develops local immunity to the common bacteria in our body and home. Within a family, common bacteria are shared. This is inevitable when meals, bathrooms, beds, linen, and clothes are shared.

Public hot tubs expose a child to bacteria from other homes. The child will not have the same local immunity to these new bacteria. I don't recommend public hot tubs to any child with problems with bladder infection.

When a child is treated with a broad-spectrum antibiotic, such as amoxicillin for an ear infection, the medication indiscriminately kills bacteria everywhere in the body; respiratory bacteria, skin bacteria, and gut bacteria. No antibiotic kills all the bacteria in the body. As such, treatment with a broad-spectrum antibiotic leaves behind the bacteria that are resistant to the antibiotic. Sometimes the resistant bacteria are more likely to cause bladder or kidney infection.

Symptoms of Isolated Bladder Infection

The symptoms of an isolated bladder infection are straightforward. The child complains that the pee hurts or burns as it comes out. The child needs to pee more often (frequency), they start to run (urgency) to get to the bathroom, and the child might be damp before they reach the toilet. The child might wet the bed at night. The mother might note an odor to the urine. Collected in a beaker, the urine looks cloudy.

Treatment of Bladder Infection

Every child with bladder infection should have a urine culture test to identify the bacteria and confirm the sensitivity of the bacteria to the common antibiotics. Based on the results of the culture an appropriate antibiotic is chosen.

My preference is to prescribe nitrofurantoin. This antibiotic is effective for ninety percent of the common bacteria that cause bladder infection. The antibiotic has less effect on respiratory and gastrointestinal bacteria and as such does not promote the development of antibiotic resistant bacteria as commonly as the other antibiotics. There is a low risk of yeast infection. Nitrofurantoin has a better side effect profile than most of the other common antibiotics. Allergic reactions are uncommon. The colour of the urine is a darker yellow than usual while the child takes the medication. Tummy upset is the only common side effect. This is more common with the suspension than the tablet or capsule formulations. The tummy upset usually develops within fifteen to thirty minutes after taking the medication. The discomfort is in the pit of the stomach just below the breast bone. Taking the medication with a meal or snack reduces the tummy upset. The discomfort is usually short-lived and resolves within half an hour. The discomfort is common with initial doses and often disappears with subsequent doses.

Prevention of Bladder Infection

Hygiene Recommendations

The girl should wipe from the front to back after each bowel movement.

The girl should promptly cleanse and rinse the genital area after a poop accident and then change into clean clothes. Children with frequent poop accidents should have a change of clothes at school so they can promptly change at school. When they return home, the child should cleanse and rinse the genital area and change into new clothes.

After each void I recommend the girl use tissue paper to mop up any drips of urine that might be retained between the labia. Chronic dampness increases the risk of a rash in the genital area.

Girls who wear a night pull up for bedwetting should remove the pull-up as soon as they wake up. They should not play in the wet pull-up.

I recommend a rinse of the genital area every morning after the child wakes. The mother might use a hand-held shower nozzle or the child can sit in several inches of water in the bathtub. The labia should be spread and water with a comfortable temperature should be rinsed for at least a minute.

I recommend showers over tub baths and I do not recommend bubble bath.

Voiding Recommendations

Encourage the child to void regularly and not to hold the urine past full.

At school the child should routinely leave class to pee and not wait for scheduled breaks. The parent should discuss leaving class with the teacher to ensure easy access to the bathroom. Voiding four times every day while at school is a good routine.

At home the child should be encouraged to void at common transition times.

Bowel Health Recommendations

Achieve bladder-friendly bowel health to prevent poop accidents and to take the pressure off the bladder.

Haemorrhagic Cystitis

Haemorrhagic cystitis is when the isolated bladder symptoms are present and the mother sees fresh blood and mucous in the urine. In haemorrhagic cystitis the inflammation in the bladder wall is severe enough to erode through a protective glycoprotein layer into the bladder muscle. Sometimes the child complains of pain in the lower abdomen (suprapubic pain). With haemorrhagic cystitis the bladder infection takes longer to heal and there is a higher relapse rate. I routinely prescribe a treatment dose of the antibiotic for one week and follow this with a lower preventative dose for a month after an episode of haemorrhagic cystitis. I arrange careful weekly follow up of the urine for a month after the child stops the antibiotic.

Kidney Infection (Pyelonephritis)

Infection in the bladder can reach the kidneys if the bacteria can navigate from the bladder up through the ureter to the kidney. Normally the bladder muscle at the junction of the ureter and the bladder contracts to prevent urine in the bladder going up to the kidney. If this mechanism fails, the urine is propelled back up to the kidney. This is counterproductive since urine in the bladder is meant to go in only one direction, out of the body through the urethra, and not back up to the kidney. When this happens, vesico-ureteral reflux is present. When vesico-ureteral reflux is present the bacteria in the bladder are propelled up to the kidney when the bladder contracts.

Kidney infections are more serious than bladder infections. The acute symptoms are more severe. There is fever and lethargy. The child might vomit. An older child might complain of back or side pain. The child looks sick. The child lays around, sleeps a lot, doesn't eat, and looks awful. If the kidney infection occurs in an infant or young child a scar might develop consequent to the kidney infection. Scars are more common in younger children because a scar is an area of the kidney that does not grow because of the damage due to the kidney infection. Kidney infection in infants and younger children has a bigger potential impact on growth because there is so much more growth yet to come. Scars are less likely after the age of eight years. After this age the kidneys are closer to adult size and the impact on growth is less. After this age there might still be damage to kidney cells in the area of infection, but a scar is less likely. Not every kidney infection develops into a scar. The reasons for this are not clearly understood. If a scar does develop there is a risk of high blood pressure in the child during adolescence or adulthood. The risk of high blood pressure is what makes kidney infection serious.

Vesico-ureteral Reflux

Vesico-ureteral reflux is diagnosed with a voiding cystourethrogram. This study requires a bladder catheter and is an emotionally and physically traumatic procedure for a child. I try to order as few of these studies as necessary. A special x-ray dye is infused into the bladder through the catheter. At a volume appropriate for the age of the child the infusion is stopped. The child is requested to pee. X-rays are taken before, during, and after voiding. Vesico-ureteral reflux is diagnosed when the x-ray images show the dye squirting back up to the kidney. Vesico-ureteral reflux is classified as mild, moderate, or severe depending on how high the dye goes up the ureter to the kidney and whether the ureter is wider than normal. The grading system has a clinical value. Mild and moderate vesico-ureteral reflux usually resolves with time, improvement in bowel health, and prevention of infection. Severe vesico-ureteral reflux might not resolve and might require treatment with a surgical procedure.

Smoldering Bladder Infection

Infection in the bladder can "smolder." Smoldering infection is likely when a mother reports "back-to-back" bladder infection or that the bladder infection comes back within a few weeks or a month after the antibiotic is finished. The symptoms of smoldering bladder infection can be subtle. There often isn't any discomfort with voiding. If a child suffers from urgency, daytime wetting, or bedwetting prior to the onset of the bladder infection, any increase in these symptoms might not be appreciated.

Sometimes the mother knows there is infection because of the smell of the urine in the toilet or in wet clothes or sheets. Sometimes the mother knows because there is a change in mood. Often, though, there are no recognizable symptoms and the bladder infection smolders unrecognized for months and even years!

Squatting is a common sign in children with smoldering bladder infection. In a squat, a child suddenly drops down from standing and sits on their heel. The child "freezes" and does not move. Mothers often remark that their child has a look of "intense concentration." Some describe this as a "deer in the headlights" look. A squat might last more than a minute. Sometimes the squat is associated with bladder pain. The child might be flushed or have tears in their eyes. The intense concentration and discomfort attests to the very high pressure in the bladder during a squat. This high pressure is not healthy for the bladder.

Squatting is a response to a sudden, overwhelming bladder contraction the child cannot suppress. The bladder contraction comes without warning. Squatting is a learned posture the child adopts to turn a soaker into modest dampness. If the mother can recollect when she first noted the squatting, this is a good way to date the onset of chronic smoldering bladder infection. Not every child who squats has smoldering bladder infection. About twenty-five percent of children who squat do so because they hold their pee until the bladder pressure is overwhelming and a contraction develops.

When bladder infection smolders over long months and years there are changes in the bladder wall. The wall gets thicker and irregular. The wall gets thicker for two reasons. One is the higher pressure when the child holds the pee past full or squats. A second reason is inflammation in the bladder wall due to smoldering infection.

Cystitis Cystica

Cystitis cystica is a chronic inflammatory condition in the bladder. The cysts are composed of submucous collections of lymphoid tissue. Cystitis cystica develops in girls with recurrent or smoldering bladder infection. In my experience the bladder infection has usually smoldered for several years before cystitis cystica develops. Why some girls develop cystitis cystica and others do not is not understood.

Once cystitis cystica develops the child is much more prone to recurrent or persistent bladder infection. The typical story is that the infection resolves while the child is treated with an antibiotic but the infection returns within weeks of stopping the medication.

The treatment for cystitis cystica is long-term preventative antibiotic therapy. The child often needs to be treated with continuous preventative antibiotic therapy for more than one year. My practice is to treat with nitrofurantoin for three months, then stop the antibiotic and closely follow the child to look for recurrence of infection. If the infection returns within a month, I treat for another three months and I continue to do this until the infection does not return. I stop the antibiotic every three months in the hope the infection will not return so that I can minimize how long a child stays on the preventative antibiotic. Frustratingly the infection often continues to return and several years of preventative antibiotic therapy might be needed.

Reasons Why Preventative Therapy is Necessary

1. With smoldering bladder infection, it might take months for the inflammation to settle down

2. It is better to prevent infection rather than accept the cycle of intermittent antibiotic treatment and frequent relapse (avoid the one step forward, two steps back pattern).

3. While on the preventative antibiotic the goal is to change basic hygiene, voiding, poop, and hydration behaviours to minimize the risk of relapse when the preventative antibiotic is eventually stopped.

Bladder wall thickness is increased in cystitis cystica. In my experience this is a good marker of the presence of cystitis cystica. The thickness of a normal bladder wall (empty with less than 5 ml of pee) should be less than 3 mm. In children with cystitis cystica I commonly see bladder wall thickness in the range of 4 to 6 mm.

The diagnosis of cystitis cystica requires a cystoscopy under anaesthesia and a biopsy of the bladder wall. If the story fits with cystitis cystica and if the bladder wall is thick, I do not recommend a cystoscopy and biopsy because the results will not change how

I treat the child. I am content to presume the child has cystitis cystica and to avoid the anaesthetic and the procedure.

Vesico-ureteral reflux is common in cystitis cystica. In one study vesico-ureteral reflux was found in 41% of children. To check for vesico-ureteral reflux requires a voiding cysto-urethrogram. I only look for vesico-ureteral reflux in children who have a history of kidney infection and especially those children who continue to develop episodes of kidney infection.

Uncommon Physical Causes of Day and Night Wetting

Neurogenic bladder

Anything that interrupts the nerves from the bladder to the spinal cord can cause a neurogenic bladder. A neurogenic bladder is a permanent disability. There is no cure. A magnetic resonant image of the lower spine is necessary to diagnose neurogenic bladder.

The most common cause is Spina Bifida, a congenital defect in the spine. Other causes include trauma to the spine (diving, trampoline, and motor vehicle accidents). Other causes include tumors and cysts that compress the nerves in the spinal cord. A tethered cord is another cause.

Children with neurogenic bladder usual have problems with bowel health, urinary tract infection, and suffer day and night wetting.

Intermittent bladder catheterization is necessary in some children to minimize wetting, help prevent bladder infection, and protect the kidneys from the effects of high bladder pressure.

Urethral obstruction

Urethral obstruction is mostly a problem in boys. The most common cause is posterior urethral valves, a congenital problem. The problem is diagnosed when a pre-natal ultrasound shows the obstruction in the kidneys (hydronephrosis) and bladder (large bladder). A surgical procedure is necessary to relieve the obstruction. Meatal stenosis is a common cause of minor ure-thral obstruction in circumcised boys. The opening at the tip of the penis is narrow. The urinary stream is narrow and often deflected upwards. A surgical procedure is necessary to relieve the obstruction.

Ectopic ureter

This is a congenital problem mostly in girls. The ureter from the kidney does not enter the bladder, but rather exits outside the body in the external genitalia, or into the bowel or vagina.

Selected Publications on Voiding Problems by Dr. Robson

Leung AKC, Robson WLM: Nocturnal Enuresis - A Common Frustration. Journal of the Singapore Paediatric Society. 1987;29:57-62.

Robson WLM: Urinary Tract Infection in Children Diagnosis and Treatment. Canadian Family Physician. 1990;36:1597-1600.

Robson WLM, Leung AKC: Children with Primary Nocturnal Enuresis. Contemporary Pediatrics. 1990;1:19-25.

Robson WLM, Leung AKC: Advising Parents on Toilet Training. American Family Physician. 1991;44:1263-8.

Leung AKC, Robson WLM. UTI in Infancy and Childhood. Advances in Pediatrics 1991;38:257-85.

Robson WLM, Leung AKC. The Circumcision Question. Postgraduate Medicine. 1992;91:237-44.

Robson WLM, Leung AKC, Hyndman CW: Vesicoureteral Reflux in Childhood. Canadian Family Physician. 1992;38:2155-62.

Robson WLM, Leung AKC: Post-Micturition Dribble Syndrome. The Hong Kong Journal of Pediatrics. 1993;10:49-52.

Robson WLM, Leung AKC, Bloom D: Daytime Wetting in Childhood. Clinical Pediatrics. 1996;35:91-98.

Robson WLM: Diurnal Enuresis. Ped in Rev. 1997;18:407-12.

Robson WLM: The after-contraction in paediatric urodynamics. British Journal of Urology. 1997;80:190-191.

Robson WLM, Leung AKC, Jackson HP, Blackhurst D. Enuresis in Children with Attention Deficit Hyperactivity Disorder. South Med J. 1997;90:503-5.

Robson, WLM, Leung, AKC: Secondary Nocturnal Enuresis, Clinical Pediatrics. 2000;39:379-385.

Robson, WLM: Nocturnal Enuresis, eMedicine Journal 2001;Volume 2, Number 9.

Robson WLM. Nocturnal Enuresis. Adv Pediatr. 2001;48:409-38.

Robson WLM. Enuresis – Pathology and Clinical Presentation. Progress in Paediatric Urology: Penwell Publishers PLC. 2002;5,117-34.

Robson WLM, Leung AKC, Van Howe R. Primary and Secondary Nocturnal Enuresis – Similarities in Clinical Presentation. Pediatrics. 2005;115:956-9.

Robson WLM, Leung AKC. Daytime Wetting. Adv Pediatr. 2006;53:323-365.

Robson WLM, Leung AKC, Thomason M: Catheterization of the bladder in infants and children. Clinical Pediatrics. 2006;45:795-800.

Robson WLM. Nocturnal Enuresis. Invited Review. Current Opinion in Urology. 2008;18:425-30.

Robson WLM. The evaluation and management of enuresis. Invited Review. New England Journal of Medicine. 2009;360:1429-36.

Tryggve Neveus, Paul Eggert, Jonathan Evans, Antonio Macedo, Søren Rittig, Serdar Tekgül, Johan Vande Walle, C. K. Yeung and Lane Robson Evaluation of and Treatment for Monosymptomatic Enuresis: A Standardization Document From the International Children's Continence Society J Urol. 2010;183:441-7.

Index Words

K

Kegel exercises, ... 67–68

kidneys, ... 33, 60, 110

    filter function, ... 71

neurogenic bladder and,

. 110

    peeing overnight and, . 72

L

labia, ... 63, 69

    relaxation of, ... 70

labial fusion, ...102

less-attentive voiders, 37–38

limbic system, . 1, 24, 26, 34,

. . . . .40, 42–43, 44

low blood sugar, ... 39–40

lumbar spine, ... 97

M

magnetic resonance imaging
(MRI), ...110

meatal stenosis, ...111

medication, ... 93, 102,
. . . . .103, 105, 108

memory, ... 7, 24, 26, 34,
. . . . .35, 41, 42, 61

morning poop,

    behaviour changing needs
    time and consistency for,
    11–12

    child's cooperation helps
    with, ... 11–12

    confrontations unhelpful
    for, ... 11–12

    enjoyable time as necessity
    for, ... 11

    as goal of bladder-friendly
    bowel health, ... 9–12

    mother's supervision as
    necessity for, . . . 10–11

    patience as necessity for,
    11

    post-breakfast toilet sitting
    as necessity for, . 10, 11

    routine in morning as
    necessity for, ... 9–10

    as soiling solution, . . . 9

Murphy, Eddie, ... 34

N

neurobiology, ...1, 24

    daytime wetting, . . 33–34

neurogenic bladder, . 97, 110

    causes of, ...110

R

S